# NO MAGIC PILL

## Be Happier and Healthier Now, Just as You Are

PETER J. BUECKER, MD

CHICAGO SPECTRUM PRESS
LOUISVILLE, KENTUCKY 40245

Chicago Spectrum Press
12305 Westport Rd.
Louisville, Kentucky 40245
502-899-1919



Printed in the U.S.A.

10 9 8 7 6 5 4 3 2 1

ISBN: 978-158374-276-1

It is with the utmost love of my profession, respect for all involved in providing healthcare, and concern for all who find themselves in need of medical services, that I offer this work. My sincere hope is that everyone who reads these pages finds value in their content.

I pray that my two beautiful daughters may grow up in a world that is happy and healthy, and where people are decent to them, and to one another.

# A Note From the Author

Thank you for your interest in my book. I am an Orthopedic Surgeon in Louisville, Kentucky, where I have been in practice since 2005. In finding that I don't often have adequate time to spend with each of my patients to teach some important concepts, I decided to write this book. It is intended to provide a personalized, intimate experience, and is meant to be a handbook to aid you in finding the happy, healthy person who resides inside each of us This book is not meant in any way to replace appropriate medical care, but to serve as a useful adjunct to it.

I believe strongly in our medical system and the people involved in it, but feel that, due to many circumstances that are inherent within our society and the system, the need for appropriate self-care (or "participatory care" as it has also been called) has never been greater. I invite you to read this book as though we were face-to-face having a conversation. Give the reflection questions some thought, close your eyes, take a couple of deep breaths, and write down the first thing that comes to mind. Also, do the exercises, and pay particular attention to how you feel as you perform them. I would encourage you to journal this as well.

This book is meant to be, more than anything, an experience. Read it and let nature take its course. From the bottom of my heart, I wish you all the happiness and healing that you seek.

*–Pete Buecker*

# Contents

# Preface

First off, let me be say, "Welcome to your new life!" The very fact that you have picked up this book is a sign that you are ready to move forward. This book is for anyone who is frustrated with being ill, overweight, in pain, stressed out, or otherwise unhappy despite multiple trips to hospitals, doctors' offices, weight loss centers, gyms, or the like. Consider this a handbook for freeing the happiest, healthiest possible version of you from whatever it is that is holding you back. Focus on how the words on the page make you feel as you read them, and how they may apply to you and your own circumstances. I wish you the best, and look forward to being your field guide on your quest.

You may have noticed that there is an epidemic of obesity, chronic illness, and generalized unhappiness in our society, and it is affecting younger and younger people. While the advances in technology, knowledge, medications, devices, and techniques in the past few decades have been remarkable, the needs of many patients continue to be unmet. This is because there is often no pill, test, or surgery available to fix what someone truly needs. As a physician, I am quite aware of the fact that much of what goes on is what I refer to as "Drive-Thru" medicine. It is very convenient to match a pill or surgery with a set of symptoms and send you on your way, with little or no attention paid to the reasons why you developed the symptoms in the first place. The real work, in my view, would be to meet you exactly where you are in your life (lifestyle choices, stress levels, home situation, work demands, cultural values, etc.), and take on whatever symptoms you are experiencing from there.

It is not that medical providers do not care or are uninterested. In fact, for most, quite the opposite is true. The reality is that the climate in which medicine is practiced in this day and age is largely prohibitive to such comprehensive care. Medical decisions are being made increasingly by insurance companies, the doctor-patient relationship has been undermined, costs are escalating out of control, and the constant threat of litigation on all sides has everyone tense. Often it seems that the odds are stacked against you, the patient, from the outset. My hope is that this book will help empower people of all shapes, sizes, and walks of life to take ownership of their health, and improve their overall state of well-being.

Many conditions that may lead you to seek medical attention are related to the fast-paced, high stress, poorly nourished lifestyles that we have been programmed by our society to lead. Please hear me when I say that whatever has led you to this point is *not your fault*. However, you have the power to *choose* where to go from here. By embracing the power of the present moment (which is all we really have anyway) and becoming aware of your body and its messages, you can truly become the happiest and healthiest possible version of yourself.

Ask yourself: How many diets have I tried and failed? How many medications do I take to relieve pain, make me less "nervous," or to help me sleep? How many hours (or dollars) a year do I spend in doctors' offices, hospitals, or getting lab tests? How many surgeries have I had, yet still feel unhappy, unwell, or in pain? How many complications, infections, or "these things always (or only) happen to me" events have I endured?

What would you do in order to be able to take control of your life, health and happiness, and become less reliant on the medical system to "fix" you? It is much easier than you could ever imagine and I promise, you *CAN* do it. In fact, you need nothing other than yourself just as you are today to do it. There is no diet, intense exercise protocol, expensive membership, special thing to buy, or anything you need to become other than you, as you currently are. In fact, **your body *naturally* wants to be healthy, happy and full of energy. All you really have to do is get out of your own way.** I am here to help you do just that.

Here is the key: cultivate awareness of yourself and surroundings, create balance in your life, and nourish your body, mind, and spirit each and every day. Be kind to yourself. The rest will take care of itself.

Your body will find its own appropriate size and shape, and you will likely find that you simply feel and function better. Granted, you may still get sick and require medication, tests, or surgery, but only if and when they are truly needed. Try it for yourself and see–you deserve it!

- *"When you are already in Detroit, you don't have to take a bus to get there."*

  *- Ram Dass*

- *"Our belief in magic solutions that may happen someday in the future keeps us from doing what we really need to do right here and right now."*

  *- Brad Warner*

- *"Every day you wake up, there is a lot more right with you than wrong."*

  *- Jon Kabat-Zinn*

## Chapter One

# DRIVE-THRU MEDICINE

You live in a fast-paced world, and you probably have come to expect results now. You have access to a great deal of information with the tap of a finger, and can shop for anything you want without leaving your home or even standing up from your chair. You can zap a meal in 30 seconds, or expect one in the time it takes to drive a car twenty feet from an intercom where it is ordered, to a window where it is retrieved. You order a pizza, and when it is not on your table going into your belly in the promised thirty to forty minutes, you have come to expect it free. You do not want to wait in a line more than three deep at the grocery, and often choose to scan your own items in order to save time. You may nearly run someone over on the way to work, in a rush to get somewhere you don't even want to be in the first place. You order your latte-du-jour in the drive-thru, because who has the kind of time to go inside? You join a gym on January 2nd each year, only to be discouraged by January 15th that you haven't lost any weight, and accept the fact that you will never lose this darned weight anyway.

Okay, maybe I am exaggerating the situation a bit, but hopefully you now are dialed into the way our society moves. You may feel tension in your body just reading and thinking about it. Everyone has experienced it. In fact, you can't avoid it. Step outside your home and you are immersed in it. Even inside your own home, you cannot escape it.

So who has the time to be sick or in pain? How many times have you thought something like "This is just a horrible time for me to be sick" or "This injury could not have occurred at a worse time"? I cannot tell you how many times these types of things are said in a typical day. Such thinking is very common, and if you have been there yourself, it is okay, everyone has. But it is important for you to realize that the way you have been conditioned to live and think is contributing to your state of dis-ease.

Attachments to the way things "should be" or how you "should feel" are a part of this. Grasping to the idea that "I never get sick" or conversely, "I always get sick" doesn't serve you well either. Illness, pain, and discontent are all normal parts of being alive, and no time for any of these is *ever* going to be convenient. The truth is that the current situation is what the current situation is, despite anything that has happened before or anything that may happen in the future. Listen to your body; it is usually trying to tell you something. Often, illness is the body's way of telling you to slow down, take better care of yourself, and to simply allow things to be as they are.

Hopefully your physician, as a fellow human, understands that you have kids, big projects at work, or are taking care of your ailing mother, and therefore are limited in what you can do to get well. You need your energy to get through the day. However, it is not fair to put all of your stress on your physician's plate and expect him to take a big bite of it during an office visit as if it were his own. He cannot in one visit, with one pill, or operation, undo something it has taken you years to develop. Nor can he expect you to turn your whole life upside down to follow some ill-conceived directive he has given you. It is likewise not fair for your provider to expect you to take some medicine that makes you feel worse than you did originally, or so sleepy and nauseated that you can't function. The key to success is open communication, realistic expectations, and balance (more on this to come).

It is perfectly appropriate for you to not like being sick or in pain. Very few people do (and we in the medical profession get deeply concerned about them). It is also perfectly appropriate for you to expect a treatment plan that works *with* your life. It may not be appropriate, however, for you to expect instant relief or a miracle cure-all.

For so many things that may be causing a symptom right now, there most often is… you guessed it… NO MAGIC PILL. Despite what the television ads or billboards say, no matter what you heard from the woman at the hairdresser's, or anything "this guy at work" may have told you, your situation is unique and unlike anyone else's.

Those of us on the other side of the equation could stand to learn a lesson about this as well. Just as patients often expect "drive-thru" service, physicians often offer it. A new pill prescribed to one person that ended all her woes will not necessarily work the same for you. Even though a particular surgeon may be the best around performing a specific procedure does not mean it is the right one for you, or that it will work for you as well as it may have for someone else. I am not, nor ever have been, an advocate for the culture of "assembly line" medicine. It is not enough to match a symptom with a pill or procedure and send you on your way. Each person is built differently, and there is a great deal of variation between people's bodies. That is why communication and honesty between physician and patient is so important.

Your physician needs to listen to your actual problem, examine you, and figure out the best way to treat you. You need to make sure you are honest about your expectations and any problems you encounter with your treatment. Always follow up with your provider after a new treatment has been started. Avoid sitting at home fretting over the fact that this one intervention did not work so you will surely never get better. There are always other options, and not every treatment works for every patient.

Realize that your care providers are human also, and therefore imperfect. They often don't like to hear that something they have offered you isn't helping. That being said, if it is not working, they need to know so they can change it for you. You have full permission to tell your healthcare provider exactly what is going on with you. It doesn't matter how she feels about it, it matters only that you are getting the care you need. She cannot hope to help you if you don't, but please, leave the judgments at home. Just because one treatment didn't do it for you does not mean your provider is "an idiot," "doesn't know anything," or "doesn't care." It simply means that a specific treatment didn't work for you. In the event that you do not feel there is a satisfactory connection between you and the provider, you may in fact need to find a new provider, and it would be perfectly appropriate to do so. Health is not always black and white. Most often there are a lot of shades of gray. Therefore, it may take some time and effort to sort out the best way to proceed with your particular problem in your particular situation.

Realize also, that healthcare providers are also under a lot of pressure from other sources. They are expected to see more and more people, therefore giving less and less time to each. They often have to make very quick decisions and institute action based on relatively limited information. At risk of beating the " drive-thru" analogy to death, they most often get you the cheeseburger just fine, but occasionally forget to hold the pickles. They are human, and have families, worries, hobbies, and like all the same types of things as you. They are doing their best, just as you do in your life. This is not an attempt to garner any sympathy, theirs is a chosen life (I personally would choose it all over again given the option). However, what is needed in the world of medical care from all parties involved are realistic expectations–a bit of understanding and a sense that we are all working toward the same goal.

Just as the preparation and enjoyment of a good home-cooked meal surrounded by your loved ones feels so much better than gulping down a cheeseburger in your car on the way to a meeting you are dreading, so it goes with your health. Constantly relying on and expecting someone else to provide a "quick fix" solution for your problem is not nearly as effective as slowing yourself down, taking good care of yourself, and being an active participant in your life and health. Your well-being is an investment that pays invaluable dividends. People often have no idea how "sick" they really are until they experience true wellness. Hopefully, this book will help you achieve at least a glimpse of that.

You only have one body for your whole lifetime. What you do with it is up to you. Be to your body what you want it to be to you. Just like a dear friend, cultivate the relationship with your body, listen to what it is telling you, recognize it is there for you from the time you are born until the time you die, and asks only for some love, kindness, and attention in return.

Ask yourself the following questions and journal your responses:

- How do I engage in "Drive-Thru" mentality in my life?

- In what ways can I communicate better with my care provider(s) regarding my health?

- What can I do to take more responsibility for my health and well-being?

- Am I willing to slow down and be engaged in my life, rather than running from "drive-thru" to "drive-thru?"

Chapter Two

# THE HOUSE THAT EGO BUILT

If you want to understand why you are the way you are and why the healthcare system is the way it is, look no further than the good old-fashioned ego.

The term is used a lot in society, and means something different to everyone who hears it. It often is thought of negatively, but the truth is everyone has an ego, so, let's define it. For the purposes of this book, the word "ego" refers to one's projected sense of self, or the "false" self. This is used mostly to protect you from things you fear, often low self-esteem, or a poorly defined sense of identity. It is a defense mechanism you have developed, usually in childhood, that ultimately inhibits you from being, or even knowing, your true self. It is a compilation of things that you believe about yourself and want others to believe as well.

For example, a man may project an image of being tough, confident and fearless, while inside he is carrying a great deal of anxiety, uncertainty, and questions about his life and value. The truth is, if he were able to simply express these fears in a healthy way, he wouldn't need to project any sort of image. He would truly *be* fearless, tough, and confident, and people would see that in an authentic way. Any action taken to build or soothe one's ego is destined to fail long term because it often is at the expense of one's truest needs or desires. The bottom line is, anytime in your life that you have done something despite your "gut" telling you to do something else, your ego has won out over the real you.

Worry not. Everyone does this in some way. It is part of being human.

When you were a child, you likely at some point internalized that you were "not okay." It may have seemed like people were constantly telling you "no" or not to do this or that. While your caregivers' intentions may have been good (i.e. to keep you safe), the message you receive is "I am not okay as I currently am. I need to be something different." Situations where the child's needs are sacrificed so those of the caregiver can be met or situations of outright abuse obviously intensify this situation significantly.

As you go through life, you are constantly trying to find the state of being or the set of items you can possess to make you "okay." You may seek it through attaining a certain educational status, job, car, vacation home, peer group, spouse, or through use of drugs, sex, gambling, or similar stimuli. The problem is, without an internal sense of being truly "okay," none of these items will ever do the job.

I bring all this up because, in general, the ego is at the root of most things in your life that lead you to be unhappy and unhealthy. Your true self would never choose to be either. Most instances where the ego acts to cause problems may be quite subtle. For instance, say that as a child you feel that your parent has treated you unfairly in some way. Everyone has experienced this, justified or not. Your true self wants to express your frustration, but maybe you have learned that to express your true feelings will cause even more problems. In an effort to "keep the peace," you bury it inside yourself and move on.

The ego here has suppressed the true self. You may even be rewarded for being "tough," "stoic," or "Mommy's 'big' boy or girl," further ingraining the behavior pattern. This leads to some level of frustration. You may go your whole life attempting to mitigate these frustrations unconsciously in various ways with all sorts of untoward consequences. If you are not aware of these frustrations, they build up, one on top of the other, like boxes in the attic of your mind. Eventually, the clutter takes over, and all sense of order is lost. This leads to anxiety and stress.

So what happens to the true self as the ego is constantly pushing it away or crowding it out? Hint: It doesn't go away.

Here is the deal: **When your ego is very close to being in line with your true self, you are happy. When your ego is in conflict with your true self, you are not. Period.**

The distance between the two often leaves you with a void inside. The further they are apart, the bigger the void. This void is often experienced as pain, anxiety, or maybe just the sense that you are "not okay." You may use all kinds of things to try to fill this void and therefore relieve the discomfort it causes, commonly food, drugs, cigarettes, alcohol, relationships, sex, television, gambling, shopping, gossiping, and the list goes on. Even things often seen as positive, such as exercise, reading books, or even education, can be used in an effort to help you avoid the reality of your true self and circumstances.

Often it is the attempt to feel good and avoid pain that leads people into all sorts of poor choices. Any relief gained from these quick fix solutions is temporary, so you try again…and again…and again–to no avail. Alternatively, you may seek to play certain roles in life to gain validation (such as pleasing, controlling, being rebellious, or ill). Again, these roles are self-created in an effort to gain a positive sense of self worth from someone or something outside of yourself. Ultimately, you can not sustain any sense of happiness or fulfillment that comes from the playing of these roles. The void persists, and you will continue to try to fill it in various ineffective ways. The failure to find what it is you are seeking leads to stress, anxiety, and/or depression, and can ultimately result in significant health-related consequences.

If you can learn to look inside of your void and fill it from within, you won't need to attempt to find fulfillment from outside of yourself at all. That is, unless you get to know and be kind to your true self, no amount of food you can eat, cigarettes you can smoke, sex you can have, booze you can drink, or "retail therapy" you can withstand will ever fill the void. Any relief obtained in these ways is temporary. The next time you experience the void, you go right back to drink from the same old well, and the cycle continues.

As you are unable to find true, sustainable inner peace, you experience stress, which may lead to anxiety, then to depression. You may experience difficulty sleeping, headaches, pain in any number of areas, and even chronic illness. Chronic stress causes elevation of stress hormones, which can lead to elevated blood pressure and heart disease; elevated blood sugar and insulin resistance (Type II Diabetes); immune dysfunction leading to infections, wound healing difficulties, autoimmune disorders; and many types of gastrointestinal disturbances and generalized susceptibility to disease, even cancer. So hopefully, you can see that resolving any conflict between the ego and your true self is a premium for your overall wellness.

Another form the ego takes is to tell you how things "should" be. Rather than focusing on what is, the mind constructs all of these fantasies about what life should or could be like or is like for other people. This is what leads almost everyone, at least at some point, to feel like "everyone else is normal, but I am not." If you have ever experienced any sense of competition, jealousy, or sense of being separate from or isolated from others for any reason, you have experienced the workings of your ego. Don't worry, *EVERYONE* experiences this, so just the fact that you have these thoughts or feelings, makes you normal. The ego is a protective mechanism and is necessary; it just sometimes oversteps its boundaries. Your job is to stop judging your inside self compared to others' outside selves. That guy at work with the sweet car and huge house may be just as doubtful inside as you, not to mention, a lot more in debt.

While your sense of "me" or "I" remains mostly stable throughout life, your body certainly changes. If you look in the mirror when you are a little kid, at age thirty, and again at sixty, the changes are obvious. This is a normal function of life. In fact, nothing in life is truly static. Everything is in a constant state of change. Why then, should you have the expectation that you should never age, feel discomfort, or "lose a step?" There are whole industries based on making you look and feel younger. Our society spends billions of dollars on resisting the natural process of aging. Could you ever be content simply with looking and feeling as you look and feel at this particular point in your life? Why should you want to wear the same suit as a celebrity on the red carpet when you can wear what *you* choose to wear to express who *you* truly are?

Another source of ego-based problems is the sense that life can be controlled or somehow manipulated to stay the way you want it.

Uncertainty is stressful, but (I hate to be the bearer of bad news) is indeed a fact of life. The harder you hang on to your sense of "normalcy" and "stability," or the way you want things to be as opposed to the way they actually are, the more stress you will experience. Learn to roll with life like riding on a raft over waves on the ocean, and you will find peace. You cannot change the hands life deals you, but you can change how you play them. Become aware of your inner world, realize that whatever emotions you experience are normal for you and perfectly valid in that particular moment, forgive yourself for your mistakes and love yourself for being "perfectly imperfect,"* and you will naturally begin to become a skilled player in this game called life. There are strategies all throughout this book to help you do this.

There is also something called the *collective ego*. This is when a whole population acts with a sense of misguided identity. Think of the world of sports; the fan base of a particular team may be very excited about having "bragging rights" after a big win over the team's rival. This euphoria often comes from a sense of superiority to the other team's fans. The illusion is that somehow "we" are better, more important, or more powerful than "them." While it is perfectly appropriate to be excited about a victory, these particular fans are deriving personal meaning from the feats of a sports team, where there is no real personal meaning to be found. The other team's fans may even feel inferior to or "less than" the victorious team's fans. Your sense of superiority or inferiority to another person in your workplace who likes another team is purely fictitious. It has no basis in reality. The truth is, you simply like different sports teams.

It would appear that the collective ego has sailed into dangerous waters in the medical world. There is often a palpable "Us versus Them" mentality. Whatever your role in the picture may be (patient, doctor, nurse, insurance company employee, attorney, hospital administrator, product vendor), there is always the opportunity to line up against another player as your perceived opponent, and it happens all the time. Again, the illusion occurs where these individuals or institutions derive personal meaning from their roles. As the various egos are engaged, tempers flare, negotiations strain, and the unifying goal of true patient care is lost. There exists a great deal of gamesmanship, mistrust, and unrealistic expectations on all sides of this. Truthfully, each of these entities simply occupies a different seat at the same table.

As a patient, you may expect your surgeon to "make you good as new." Frankly, unless you have just been born, you are not new. It is the surgeon's task to make you as well as you can be for the state of health in which you currently find yourself. Your task is to take responsibility for whatever that state may be and take good care of yourself. That being the case, your surgeon may still promise to make you "perfect" again, as there certainly is competition in the marketplace, and thus a premium on pleasing both patients and referring physicians. Communication between the physician and patient with regard to appropriate expectations is crucial.

Likewise, it is not fair for your physician to tell you to lose 100 pounds if you want to feel better if he doesn't understand your life circumstances, how you developed the problem with your weight to begin with, or offer you any kind of realistic way of going about losing the weight. Insurance companies threaten to penalize physicians for various aspects of their practice patterns, limit services to patients, expect premium service at discount prices, all the while posting huge profits and multimillion dollar bonuses for their executive officers. Physicians and hospitals are in constant competition with other physicians and hospitals to get a bigger and bigger piece of the proverbial pie. Drug companies market on television trying to convince you that taking the "little purple pill" or that sitting in a bathtub on a beach with your dearly beloved will take away all your troubles. Trial lawyers have created a standard of perfection that keeps *everyone* on edge, and leads to literally billions of dollars in excess cost by way of tests, office visits, medications, procedures, and insurance premiums.

This is of course a gross generalization of the problems, but in many ways, it would appear that control has been lost. The ego-based needs for money, power, and control have led the system into this situation, and ultimately, the patients are the ones who often get lost in the shuffle.

If all involved were listening to their true selves and could begin to understand that their deepest human nature is to be happy, loving, and compassionate to one another, the system would actually serve to heal and nurture the way it was intended. All involved parties could also stand to realize that people, at an elemental level, are basically the same. Each of us wants to be happy, loved, well, safe, and to have a meaningful life. Just because your physician is your physician and you are the patient, does not mean you are any different. In fact, tomorrow she could be in need of your services and the roles would be very much reversed.

Imagine a system where physicians and patients could interact as mutually empowered individuals working together to achieve the highest level of well-being for the patient, patients would be active participants in their own care, insurance companies could truly concern themselves with helping provide access to the system for those who need it, and lawyers could provide a safeguard to ensure safety and equality of the care provided. To get there, all involved parties need to realize that they are all in this together, and stop fanning the flames of division between them.

By learning to watch the movements of the ego, understand the ways in which it shows itself, and not allow it to be in total control (on autopilot, as it often is) people as a whole would be much happier and healthier.

Listen to and be kind and compassionate to your true self. Be to others what you want to receive in return. If you want your doctor to be nice to you, be genuinely nice to her. If your niceness is not returned, try compassion as a response; you have no idea what is going on in her life. She may be in a great deal of pain and in that case, you may have a great deal more in common than you ever imagined.

Ghandi said "Be the change you wish to see in the world." Jesus offered us "do unto others as you would have done unto you," and the Buddha told us that anger would never be defeated by anger, only by love and compassion. All of these involve bringing the ego in line with your best interest, being true to yourself, and experiencing the inner peace and wellness that follow.

Ask yourself the following questions and journal your responses:

- What are some times that I have sacrificed my true self in the face of my ego?

- How cluttered is my mental attic? Do I have difficulty thinking, making decisions, or sleeping at night because my mind is always running?

- How does my inner void affect the choices I make?

- What do I do to ease the pain when I feel down or emotionally injured?

- Can I accept the fact that my true feelings are perfectly valid despite what I may have been taught about feeling or expressing emotion?

- What can I do to honor my true wants and desires, and to feel more grounded in just being myself?

- Can I let go of my need to be something other than I am?

- Can I learn to accept myself for who I am and my circumstances for what they are? Can I learn to ride the waves of my life as they unfold in each moment?

Try the exercise below to practice nurturing your true self. Reflect on it for a few minutes, then journal what you experienced. If this makes you feel uncomfortable, that is okay. In fact, the more difficult this is for you, the more you definitely need to do it and really process what you felt. I adapted this from an exercise conducted by Jack Kornfield as part of a web-based program called "Mindfulness and the Brain."** I tried it this way and found it quite powerful. In his version, the exercise was done with another individual, and I would encourage you to try it that way as well. I hope you find it impactful.

> Stand in front of a mirror, about the same distance you would if you were talking face to face with someone. Sitting with a hand held mirror can also work. Look at yourself. Imagine this is someone you've never met before. Look at your face and take a moment to really take in what you see. Notice the expression. Do you know this person? Do you like, dislike, or feel neutral about this person? Do you wish something were different about the face you see? Note any feelings that arise inside yourself and any thoughts that come to mind.
>
> Now, look deeply into your own eyes. Realize that there are thoughts going on in that mind. Take a moment to consider the sadness, hurt, and pain experienced by this person. Think about how you would comfort this individual if you could. Imagine looking into these eyes as a five year-old seeing sadness. What would you say to or do for this child to let her know that it is okay to be sad, but that she is loved and supported, knowing that all she really wants is to be happy, playful and free.
>
> *Close your eyes and take a couple of deep breaths.*
>
> Now look back into the eyes in the mirror. Imagine these eyes again as a child, but now the child is experiencing great joy. Maybe he has just opened his most treasured Christmas present or scored the winning run in a ballgame. Note his delight and excitement. Think of how happy you are for him. How would you celebrate with him and let him know how proud you are of him? You may actually say something aloud to him at this point.
>
> *Close your eyes and take a couple of deep breaths.*

> Look back into your eyes one last time. What do you see now that is different than a few moments ago when you first looked? Have they softened? Are there tears? Is there peace and contentment, or is there anger and resentment. Know that anything you are experiencing at this moment is normal and perfectly appropriate. Allow yourself to really feel it. If you need to say something to the person in front of you, say it out loud. If you would like to write a letter to this person, do that. Before leaving the mirror, if you feel comfortable, look deeply into your eyes and say "I love you for all that you are and all that you are not," or something similar that is personal to you.

This can be a very powerful exercise, and one I would encourage you to come back to a few times as you work your way through this book. If strong feelings arise that you don't know how to process, I would encourage you to seek the help of a therapist. There is a notion in this country that only people with "real problems" or who are "crazy" seek help with their mental health. Let me break it to you gently: we ALL have "real problems" and are at times *all* a bit crazy. The healthiest thing to do is to get help if you feel in any way that you need it. A lot more people do it than you would ever know, and there is nothing taboo about doing so.

Also, moving forward, realize that everyone you meet is, in some way, that five year-old child you saw in the mirror. We all carry wounds, joys, and memories from our past and dreams for our future. There is no one out there who is any more or less "normal" than anyone else. We are all simply walking around in different states of ego imbalance and with voids of all different shapes and size. So, the next time you encounter someone who is being difficult, imagine that five year old stomping on the ground in anger, or with tears of sadness from being let down or disappointed. You may feel something very peculiar inside that is different than the way you would normally react to a difficult person. You may feel it along with your normal reaction, which is your ego. The other feeling is compassion.

Recommended Reading:

| | |
|---|---|
| John Bradshaw | *Homecoming* |
| Thomas Harris | *I'm OK, You're OK* |
| Jon Kabat-Zinn | *Coming to Our Senses* |
| | *Wherever You Go, There You Are* |
| Alice Miller | *The Drama of the Gifted Child* |
| Don Miguel Ruiz | *The Four Agreements* |
| | *The Fifth Agreement* |
| | *The Mastery of Love* |
| Eckart Tolle | *A New Earth* |
| | *The Power of Now* |

---

* I love this term and quoted it from Pia Mellody's *The Intimacy Factor.*

** The original exercise was part of a Sounds True webinar entitled "Mindfulness and the Brain," featuring Daniel Siegel and Jack Kornfield.

## Chapter Three

# YOU ARE AS YOU ARE

A significant part of what ails us or causes us to suffer is our attachment to a certain way of feeling or being. Of course, every one wants to be well and pain-free all of the time, but that is not realistic. Illness, pain, and discontent are as much a fact of life as birth and death. It is just part of the deal, folks. So, since it can not be avoided, why not learn to roll with it or even (dare I say) embrace it. Often it is in times of stress and adversity that the most can be learned about oneself. The same could be said for illness and pain. It is often the desire to avoid discomfort or outright anger at having discomfort that causes the most problems. Letting it be, learning about it, and listening to what it is telling you can be quite revealing. Being mindful of your inner world is the best means to do just that.

Mindfulness means having nonjudgmental awareness of the present moment, as it truly exists. It is a way of life. Better yet, it is a way of being. You may have all sorts of ideas of how a particular moment should be, how you would like it to be, or what this guy or that woman should be doing. But the fact is, in that moment, things are exactly as they are. This seems pretty obvious, but the ego has a very hard time with the concept. You naturally want things to be the way that best serves your needs, regardless of the way they actually are. For instance:

> When you walk into the bank, you want to get to a teller, get your business done and get out of there. If you walk in, and

> there is one teller with four people waiting in line, you may get upset at the bank's poor planning, bad customer service, or even at the other people in line ("Don't these people have somewhere else they could be? Don't they have lives?"). This does no one any good, because the obvious fact is, there is one teller with four people waiting in line. So, you have some choices: You can leave, you can wait and be angry or resentful, or you can accept the moment for what it is, complete your business, and go about your day. Part of the reason you may feel angry in such a situation is that you have a lot of other things to do, may be running late for a meeting, or are just outright impatient. Regardless of your issues, it really doesn't concern the other five individuals in the scenario. They all have their own concerns, and yours, frankly, are yours and no one else's. You are likely best served by accepting the situation for what it is, realizing that all these people are in the same boat as you, and dealing with the situation as it is.

This is a concrete example of an isolated incident. We all have these moments. Do not worry if you have done this, as everyone has. But what if the situation is more chronic? What if you have chronic low back pain, which is a very common condition? Maybe you got this from a work-related accident years ago and haven't known a day without pain since. You would have every right to feel resentful, thinking that you should have never been on that job in the first place or why couldn't this have happened to someone else? You may also be depressed about the prospects of living the rest of your life with this pain. "*If only I could go back and change things…*"

All of this is a very normal reaction to such a situation. But, the fact is, you *were* on that job and *did* get this injury and it *did* happen to you, not someone else. The past is the past, and therefore, cannot be changed. The future has not yet happened, and therefore, there is no way to know if you will continue to be in pain, or what may transpire. In fact, the human mind tends to get anxious about the future and, most often, anticipates things being a whole lot worse than they actually turn out to be. You are not alone if you do this; it is, in fact, part of the human survival mechanism. Simply being aware of this can help decrease your overall anxiety level.

The only moment you have any ability to directly impact is the present one. Actually, if you think about it, life is nothing more than a constant flow of present moments. Our minds hold on to the past in many ways, but the fact is, once the moment has passed, it has passed. You may think of a time that your favorite team won a championship, for instance. That is a great feeling isn't it? But it is short lived, because you will immediately start thinking about whether or not your team can win it again and how long it may take and how you hope this team or that team doesn't win the next championship, and on and on and on. Already the present is in the past and you have become consumed with the future. This is how the majority of people live their lives, and it takes its toll.

Constant ruminating about past events and/or fear of things that may be yet to happen can lead you into a state of chronic stress. As previously mentioned, this can have all kinds of disastrous effects on your health. There are a lot of good resources on the specifics of the chronic stress response (see below), but basically, in any situation of stress the body activates the "fight or flight" response.

For instance, if you are walking home at night and a man in a mask jumps out from behind a building, your heart starts racing, your breathing gets fast, you get some "butterflies" in your stomach, and you take off running. In that instant, cortisol and adrenaline were released from your adrenal glands after a signal from your brain to turn on this response. Your heart rate, blood pressure, blood sugar, and respiration increased; blood flow to your muscles increased and the activity of your immune, reproductive, and gastrointestinal systems all but ceased. This series of changes is quite important when faced with an imminent threat and a need to move quickly to survive.

However, chronic stress leads to a prolonged "fight or flight" response. This can go on for years, or even a lifetime if left unattended. The same physiological changes occur as above, but over a much longer period of time. What results are conditions like reflux (GERD or "heartburn"), obesity, high blood pressure, heart disease, diabetes, low thyroid activity, generalized anxiety disorder (which may also lead to depression), headaches, various types of chronic musculoskeletal pain, and immune dysfunction (including autoimmune diseases, wound healing difficulties and even cancer) to name a few.

Jon Kabat-Zinn and Saki Santorelli at the University of Massachusetts have been pioneering in the field of stress reduction for over 30 years. Programs based on their work have popped up all over the world with great success. Mindfulness is the crux of these programs (Mindfulness Based Stress Reduction or MBSR). Briefly stated, the focus of this program is the development of moment to moment awareness of one's body, thoughts, sensations, and emotions in an effort to reduce stress and become more at peace with one's self and circumstances (there is more on this in the next chapter).

I would challenge you to consider that you are truly unique. There has never been, nor will ever be, anyone else exactly like you. Your history is your history, and your future is your future. You have only this life to live in this particular body. So why spend it in so much stress and discontent? Happiness, laughter, love, kindness, and compassion have so many health benefits and provide such a nice alternative to distress and the associated feelings of separation, isolation, and anger. Whatever has happened in the past has served to bring you to this point, for whatever reason. Embrace this. Embrace yourself in this moment *exactly* as you are. Take another look at yourself in the mirror and remind yourself of who that person is and where he or she came from. Take inventory of who that person is today and where you would like for him or her to go from here. Remember, the future has not happened yet, and therefore it is completely modifiable. It is okay to plan and have dreams and goals, as long as your attention remains predominantly in the present moment and is not consumed with how things may one day be for you.

By learning to accept, have compassion for, and, yes, love yourself for exactly who you are, regardless of anything that has happened in your past or may be going on currently, the void will start to fill. Whether you realize it yet or not, just by getting to this point in this book, you are well on your way.

Try the following mindfulness exercise to begin familiarizing yourself with yourself, as you are today. This can be very eye-opening if you have never done something like this before. Take note of what you feel, think, and experience. You may also wish to journal this. You can do one part, read the next instruction, and continue, record yourself reading this slowly and follow along; or have a trusted someone read this to you. The most important thing is to find what works best for you. After all, this is all about getting to know yourself better.

Find a seat in a comfortable chair where you can sit for an uninterrupted 15-20 minutes. Make sure your back is well supported and your feet are planted firmly on the ground. Rest your arms with your hands on your lap or resting on the arms of the chair. Once you are settled, close your eyes. Start by just sitting quietly for a minute or two. Take a couple of deep breaths, and blow out the tension of the day.

Now, bring your attention to the fact that you are breathing. There's no need to alter or count your breaths, or manipulate them in any way. Just breathe in and out naturally. Try breathing into and out of your belly (diaphragmatic breathing), allowing your belly to rise as you breathe in, and fall as you breathe out. Place your hand on your belly to feel this if you aren't sure whether or not you are doing this correctly. Try this for a minute or two.

Notice that as you do this, that your mind will wander. When this happens, acknowledge what it is you're thinking about and return your attention back to your breathing. Do this for a couple of minutes and notice how you feel as you do this.

Next, turn your attention to your body and any sensations you may be feeling. Become aware of any tingling, sensitivity, pain, tension, or whatever else you may experience. Start by turning your awareness to your feet, slowly work up your legs, to your knees, and then to the thighs and hips. Next, feel into your stomach, chest, and then your back noting any areas of tension or discomfort. Next, turn your awareness to your hands, forearms, and elbows, working slowly up to your shoulders. Next, sense your neck, face, head, and scalp. What do you notice as you do this? Just as in the breathing portion, if your mind wanders off, gently turn your attention back toward the body part you last focused on, and then continue. How are you feeling now?

Next, turn your awareness to sounds. Note any sounds coming from your body. You may hear your pulse, or sounds from your stomach, throat, or nostrils. See what sounds arise from your immediate surroundings, or even outside. Just note how these affect you as you notice them.

Finally, open up your awareness to whatever arises. Start with your breath, and then open yourself to your sensations, sounds, thoughts and feelings. As thoughts come up, see if you can simply observe them and let them go as opposed to getting caught up in them. As a thought arises, note any feelings in your chest, belly, or other areas that may accompany it. After noting these feelings, observe them, then let them go, returning to a state of awareness of your inner and outer worlds, just as they are in the present moment.

When you are ready, open your eyes, and note how you feel. How does the room look to you compared to how it did before you started this exercise? What kind of thoughts came up in your mind while you were doing this? Treat yourself to this type of exercise every day for 15-20 minutes as a "time out" from everyday life. As you are comfortable, stretch out the time spent to 30, 45, or even 60 minutes.

What you have just done is a basic type of sitting meditation. Repeating this exercise daily for a period of time will help you really start settling into yourself. You will gain understanding of how your thoughts move, how your emotions interact with your thoughts, and how your body feels when this happens. Also, note that you can observe your thoughts and emotions without getting attached to them.

As you learn to do this in meditation, see how this works in your daily life. As encounters arise, allow the associated thoughts and emotions to arise and pass without getting "caught" by them. Be aware that the average thought lasts only a few seconds, and the average emotion about a minute and a half. That is, unless you attach to them, then they can go on for very long periods of time. If you do get attached, don't worry. Just like in the meditation, note that you got "caught," forgive yourself, and try again next time. This is a way of practicing love, forgiveness, and compassion for yourself. Your health and wellness will thank you.

Recommended Reading and/or listening:

| | |
|---|---|
| Thich Nhat Hanh | *The Miracle of Mindfulness* |
| Rick Hanson | *Stress-proof Your Brain* |
| Mark Hyman | *Ultramind Solution* |
| Jon Kabat-Zinn | *Full Catastrophe Living* |
| | *Mindfulness for Beginners* |
| Saki Santorelli | *Heal Thyself* |
| Esther Sternberg | *The Balance Within* |

If you would like to try a guided sitting meditation, there are many out there. I would recommend starting with one of the following:

Jon Kabat-Zinn "Guided Mindfulness Meditation" (Disc Three: Sitting Meditation)

Jack Kornfield "Guided Meditation" (Sitting Meditation)

## Chapter Four

# THE IMPORTANCE OF BALANCE

Now that you are working toward the right state of mind for achieving holistic wellness (body, mind, and spirit), let's start talking strategy. You have likely heard some variation of the old phrase "all things are okay in moderation." I would like to tweak that a bit. If you are engaged in a lot of bad health habits, but all in moderation, the overall effect is still bad for your health. Think of your health as a bank account. If you add up a bunch of withdrawals, without some deposits along the way, you are going to go broke. But who wants to live a life where all we do is save, save, save, and never spend, right? It is much safer to withdraw money from your account as long as you are putting an equal amount or better back in. As long as you can pay your bills and care for yourself and your family, then you can spend a little on yourself every once in a while.

A similar concept applies to your health and wellness. The key is balance. It is okay to eat a piece of carrot cake every once and again if you are otherwise eating in a healthy way, and are engaged in sufficient physical activity to burn off some of those calories. It is normal to have stress in life, sometimes quite a lot of it. So balance that with some good rest and relaxation, particularly when your body is telling you that you need it. Work can be very demanding, and you may spend a lot of hours there. So make sure there is relatively equivalent time, or at least energy, spent on your hobbies, family and other important relationships. If you like to watch television at night, watch what you really want to see, then balance that with some time spent in reading, doing puzzles, or otherwise stimulating your brain.

**True wellness is not about turning your life upside down in an effort to lose weight, become healthier, or to make yourself somehow different. That almost never works long-term. It's about working *WITH* your life, being present to whatever is currently happening, and focusing on establishing balance.**

To do this, you have to learn to pay attention to your life. There is no substitute for awareness when it comes to taking yourself where you want to go.

In my experience, if you want to achieve wellness of your body, mind, and spirit, the following factors in your life need to be in balance:

- Spirituality
- Stress
- Brain Stimulation
- Body
- Food
- Family and Intimate Relationship
- Work
- Social Interaction and Friendships

Notice the order in which I have presented these items. This may seem strange to you at first glance. You most likely have not been programmed to live in this fashion. However, true balance starts with you. Only when you are caring for yourself can you truly engage with others effectively. If you learn nothing else from this book, focus on developing present-moment awareness, and being conscious of your level of balance in these areas, each day, in your own life. I would encourage you to take daily inventory of your life regarding these factors as presented, in this order. After a while, it will become natural.

Achieving balance does not necessarily mean spending equal time on all of these factors, I'm not sure anyone could ever accomplish that. It is more about how you focus your attention and priorities. I should also note that the level of each that achieves the right balance for one person will be different than for others. That is why awareness is so important. Figure out what works for you by listening to your body and your inner self as you learned in the previous chapters. You will find that you will settle into a groove that feels right for you. It doesn't matter what another person's balance is; what matters is your balance. Remember, you are unique and special unto yourself. ***Be who you truly are, not who someone or everyone else wants or expects you to be.***

A word about emotions is warranted before moving on to a discussion of the eight factors. If you think of the aforementioned factors as the building blocks of your life, then your emotions are the glue that holds them all together. If your emotions are off kilter, so it will be for the rest of you.

Emotions are often the body's response to thoughts. Please hear me when I say, *There is nothing wrong with experiencing emotions.* In fact, you may go through several of them in the course of an average day, and nothing could be more human. It is the way you relate to your emotions that causes the problems.

You may have been taught not to express, or even feel, emotions. Often this is done from a place of love. As a parent you may say to your child who is crying, "Don't be sad." What you are intending to convey is, "I don't want you to be sad because it hurts me to see you that way." What the child hears is, "Don't be sad; it's not okay to be sad." Alternatively, you may say, "Only babies cry, are you a baby?" This encourages the child to stifle her emotions. Though she is a very young child now, she will carry this into adulthood where it may cause all sorts of disturbances in her life. Most often, the inability to adequately express emotions leads to chronic anxiety and/or depression, both of which are highly prevalent in today's society.

Only by learning to recognize and express your emotions as they arise can you begin to bring them into balance. The meditation exercise from the previous chapter can help you begin to see how thoughts and emotions connect. By realizing that an emotion is a response to a thought, you can learn to witness them as they occur, let them be, then let them go without getting attached to them. You can stop judging yourself for having them, and as your emotions come into balance, many other pieces of the puzzle will start to fall into place.

## Spirituality

While I am no spiritual master or guru, what I can say on the subject is, whether or not you are a particularly religious or spiritual individual, what is required for a truly balanced and meaningful existence is some sense of connection to something greater than yourself. Whether for you this means God, unified consciousness, nature, or humanity itself, it is important to be connected to something. That is, developing a *real* connection in a way that you feel that your very essence, soul, or true self is a part of the bigger picture of humanity or beyond. This of course, needs to be in balance with your greater sense of yourself and your level of balance with regards to all of the other factors in your life.

Regardless of what it is, your spirituality infuses itself into all that you do and all that you are. Viewing yourself as being a single stitch in a much broader cloth allows you to keep your life in perspective. It helps dissolve your preoccupation with "I" or "me" and the stress involved with maintaining the ego's illusion of separation (which in turn causes its own level of anxiety). You realize that you are a vital part of the world around you. Attending to yourself from this perspective affords you the opportunity to nourish and care for yourself from a position of responsibility and love, which greatly enhances your ability to bring the other necessary components of your life into balance.

## Stress

The next chapter is all about managing your stress. For now, let's just say that stress creates significant roadblocks to the expression of your true self, contributes to your overall level of anxiety, and is one of the key contributors to illness in our society. That being said, finding healthy outlets for your stress is critical to achieving balance.

I notice that when asked how they relieve stress, a lot of people say they watch television, read books, or work out. While these may at times be relaxing, I tend to see them more as distraction. It is akin to a child burying his head in the pillow and thinking you can't see him. Stress is the same way. Burying your head in distraction does not get rid of the stress; it just allows you to avoid it for a while.

Stress is like a volcano. If there is regular release of its energy in effective ways (e.g. the geysers like "Old Faithful" at Yellowstone National Park), it doesn't erupt. But if no outlet is available, eventually the pressure builds and disaster occurs. For you, this could be depression, high blood pressure, high blood sugar, chronic pain, heart attacks, strokes, cancer, or other serious disease states.

The key is finding ways to truly vent the stress. Balancing your emotions through meditation and/or journaling is a great start. Mindful movement (e.g. yoga, qi gong, tai chi), cardiovascular exercise working the large muscle groups (walking, jogging, stationary cycling), or getting a massage all provide excellent avenues to release muscle tension associated with stored stress.

Use caution in working out to relieve stress. Make sure you are relaxed, and in a good place mentally and emotionally before exercising. If you perform rigorous physical activity while actively stressed, you may only train your muscles to hold and store the stress, and this can lead to pain, injury, or worse. By learning to read your body's signals, you can learn to identify stress and explore ways to release it before it can take hold of your health and well-being.

## Brain Stimulation

One thing I have seen time and time again in my personal and professional life that never ceases to amaze me, is how quickly a person will decline in health when she stops stimulating her mind. How many times have you seen someone retire from a long career only to completely fall apart mentally, emotionally, and physically? There is all sorts of research on the positive effects of brain stimulation, including delaying or preventing the onset of dementia. Your brain is a "use it or lose it" structure. I highly recommend that you use it.

Brain stimulation may mean very different things to different people. Learning new skills, information, a new language, taking up art, music, crafts, working crossword puzzles, or playing chess are all examples of ways to keep your brain healthy and engaged. Watching your diet, balancing the use of intoxicants such as alcohol, eliminating cigarettes and drugs from your life, and meditating on a regular basis are all great strategies for optimizing the health and function of your brain. Don't sacrifice your brain for anything. Make this a priority. It is a wondrous and beautiful structure, more complex and mysterious than you can ever imagine. It holds the keys to everything.

## Body

You have heard it said, and it is true, your body *is* your temple. Your body is what carries you around throughout your life. Treat it as such. You have been gifted your body from your parents, and theirs before them, and theirs before them and so on. Your body is a continuation of your family throughout time, so it truly is divine. By respecting and nurturing your body, you are paying tribute to the gift you have been given by your ancestors.

Your body requires certain things to work properly. First, it needs fuel, which includes appropriate amounts of protein, fat, and carbohydrates (yes, it needs fat). It needs a number of vitamins and minerals to help keep the factory running smoothly, and it also needs activity. Moving your body is important, as this keeps blood flowing to your brain and other critical organs, and keeps your heart beating strong and efficiently. It keeps your muscles healthy, and helps keep the energy flow in your body–you guessed it–balanced!

Your body also needs love. If you love your body and treat it with respect, it will do the same for you. Not that you won't get sick or have problems, but your relationship with it, even in illness, will be more healthy. It is definitely worth pursuing.

Balance the needs of your body with those of your mind, heart, and spirit. Understand your body for what it is, as it is. Be loving and compassionate to it, and it will return the favor. Exercise or move because you choose to, not to attain some shape or size that is totally unnatural to you. Get to know your body by listening to what it is telling you (meditation such as the sitting practice in the last chapter will really help). Learning to read your body's signals (such as food cravings) will help you understand what it wants and how to take care of it. Don't overwork your body without balancing it with rest and relaxation. If you tend to hold stress in certain areas, focus on these during the body scan portion of meditation. Try getting a massage at least once in a while, and have your therapist focus specifically on these areas. Treat yourself. You are totally worth it.

## Food

In our society we eat…and we eat…and eat. Eating is often associated with love. I cannot visit my grandmother without getting fed. No matter how much I resist, I know it is futile, and I eat because for her, it is a sign of love. This is completely the wrong reason to eat, yet the fact is that most eating done in our society is conditioned and emotional. We eat because we are supposed to eat. When we feel sad, we eat. When we feel happy we eat. When we are bored, we eat. When we watch television, we eat. We snack at work and munch at ballgames, movies, and meetings. We eat constantly. The way we relate to food in our country is completely out of balance, and one of the main reasons for our epidemic of obesity.

By understanding your motivations to eat, your association of certain foods with certain emotional states, and becoming aware of those states before giving into them, you can start to bring your relationship with food into balance. Most diet and exercise regimens fail to address this properly, thus their high failure rate. In fact, if you are stressed about losing weight, compulsively weighing in and anxious about whether or not you are doing enough exercise or eating the right things at the right times, keeping food journals, and beating up on yourself when you "mess up," you will actually gain weight, regardless of how faithfully you follow your trainer's or nutritionist's instructions. The chronic stress response that this behavior pattern generates leads to poor digestion, diminished nutrient absorption, overeating, and weight gain. Unless your emotional self is in balance, you will be defeating yourself from the outset.

If instead, you begin to have compassion for yourself, learn to forgive yourself for your imperfections and love yourself as you are, whatever shape or size you are, you will eat to nourish rather than to soothe (or abuse) yourself. Your body will take its most natural form, and you will feel and look better than you ever have before. You may choose to be more active because you will feel like being active, and will choose to eat healthier, because you will feel better when you do. You will wake up to find yourself in a whole new, healthier relationship with yourself, your body, and food.

## Family

There can be no greater source of happiness than a rich and meaningful family life. It can also be a great source of stress. Raising children, maintaining your marriage, caring for an ailing parent, sparring with siblings or in-laws, and all of the other things that go with family life can definitely start to weigh on you. It can be easy to lose yourself in all the hustle and bustle of daily family life, but I will encourage you not to do that. Appropriately caring for yourself is a gift of love to yourself and your family. If you are not attending to your own needs, you will not be at your best attending to those of others. That is why balance is so critical.

Managing your stress, stimulating your mind, nourishing your body, and staying active are great ways to offset the difficulties of family life. Utilize your resources to make it happen. The value of taking care of yourself cannot be overstated. Negotiate childcare duties with your spouse. Work with your siblings to take shifts with your ailing parent, or even hire a sitter or home nurse. Allow yourself room to truly relax, eat well, sleep, and be rejuvenated. If you are constantly stressed out and exhausted, you will get sick, and then what service are you to anyone?

This is YOUR life, not anyone else's. You may have been taught that to attend to our own needs is selfish. This could not be further from the truth. By keeping yourself refreshed, healthy, and energetic, you can truly give of yourself fully without running yourself into the ground. What a gift that is to those who need you. Your family members are people first and foremost. They have the same potential as you to take care of themselves. Allow them to explore this. Killing yourself to take care of another who is perfectly capable of taking care of himself or herself does neither of you any good. Be your own advocate. Care for yourself. Choose to offer yourself to others. There is no rule that says you *have* to do anything for anyone. You should give of yourself by choice from a place of love and compassion, not from a sense of obligation or guilt. Being loving brings love, while being obliged brings resentment. Again, stay aware of now and choose your life, moment by moment by moment.

## Work

It has been established that you live in a fast paced, high stress society. You work too much, rest too little, and your body and mind pays the price. If you are fortunate enough to be able to work, your job likely takes up the largest chunk of your time in the course of a typical day.

Despite how you may feel about your job, it is quite beneficial on many levels. First and foremost, working allows you to support yourself financially. Without money, it is very hard to live, since shelter, food, and life's other comforts obviously do not come for free. Beyond this, however, the work environment provides important opportunities for social interaction with co-workers, customers, and others you encounter throughout the day. It may offer you important outlets to express yourself and tap into your creativity. You may find yourself challenged or stimulated in all kinds of ways, positive and negative.

Regardless of the type of job you have or the atmosphere in your workplace, opportunities for personal growth abound. You may choose to view good and difficult times at work as a chance to learn something important about yourself; how you react, respond, feel or choose to act in a situation can tell you a lot about the workings of your ego, emotions, and true self.

Balancing your work with the rest of your life can be a huge challenge. This makes it all the more important to really focus on doing this. For instance, work is often the source of a great deal of stress. This may be physical, mental, time management, or family-related stress. It is important to offset this stress in some way. Carrying it with you without an appropriate outlet takes its toll on your body and well-being.

People tend to make poor food choices at work, and often may multi-task while eating. This leads to all sorts of problems. This will be explored in more depth in the next chapter. Suffice it to say, eating bad food in a hurry while doing multiple tasks at the same time does not serve your body well.

Time at work also means time away from family, friends, or others who may be important to you. When you do get home, you may be consumed with thoughts or feelings about the day at work, stress about upcoming projects and deadlines, or may even live in a chronic state of falsely associating your identity with your job. This leads to problems, as you are not your job, you are who you are. Your job is what you do. When you identify yourself with your job, you lose track of who you really are. When you lose track of who you are, you suffer.

Balance is the key. Staying in touch with your true self and remaining focused in the present moment can allow you to enjoy your work, be present for your family when you are home, and allow you to appropriately manage your stress and care for your body. Remember, it is not the quantity of time that maintains the balance in your life, it is the quality of the focus and effort. The freedom and energy that come from living in balance will allow you to be at your best at work, yet allow you to also be "in the zone" with your family when you return home. You will stop taking out your work frustrations on your spouse and kids, sleep better, feel refreshed when you get up, have more energy throughout the day, and your life will take on new meaning.

## Social Interaction/Entertainment

Humans are social animals. We need love, support, laughter, camaraderie, and affectionate touch to thrive. Some of us, however, use socializing as a way to avoid loneliness, emptiness, or the pain that results from an internal void. In this case, balancing social time with self-nurturing (like the exercises presented in previous chapters) will help you feel better in your own skin, and make social interaction more meaningful and less anxiety provoking.

Socializing from a place of love within yourself as opposed to socializing in an effort to seek affirmation or validation from other people is the name of the game. If you are seeking something from others that you don't have inside you already, you will always be disappointed. It is not fair to your friends or family to expect them to provide you with happiness, purpose, or meaning. You have to find that in yourself. Once you have found your own internal fulfillment, be loving toward your friends. This will bring the love from them that you seek. It requires minimal effort, but the return is amazing. Leave your ego at home, and offer your friends and loved ones the real you. This is the basis of the popular saying "Love like you've never been hurt," since once hurt, your ego will try to defend against future pain. Let it be, recognize life for what it is, and choose to love fully and deeply. If you get hurt, get up and do it again. You won't regret it.

It is also important to balance social and entertainment endeavors with time spent with family, stimulating your brain, and exploring your inner self. They are all important for your overall well-being. Stay present when socializing, and see others for who they truly are. Identify how you feel about them and why. Prioritize relationships that elevate your true self and awareness to a higher level. Avoid gossip and harmful talk; speak and act from a place of love, kindness, and compassion. Your heart will grow, your spirit will be light, and your health will benefit.

In summary, there are multiple factors involved in living a balanced life. It all starts with gaining awareness of your thoughts and emotions. Bringing the eight key factors of your life into balance based on your level of focus and attention will help you live happier, healthier, and more freely.

Perform the following exercise to help you achieve balance in your life:

- Draw a large circle on a sheet of paper. Imagine this is a pie with eight slices. Each slice represents one of the eight factors of balanced living. Draw the pieces of the pie with each being a size relative to how you would like to allot your time and energy in an ideal world. This is your "Ideal Priorities Pie."

- Next, draw another circle the same size, and this time, size the pie pieces based on how you actually involve yourself with the eight factors in your everyday life. This is your "Actual Priorities Pie." Compare the two. What stands out? Are there any surprises? What can you do to bring the two closer together?

- Finally, draw a circle with the eight pieces sized to reflect what you feel you can realistically achieve. This is your "Balanced Life Pie." When done, place this on your refrigerator or tape it to your bathroom mirror or similar location where you will see it everyday and be reminded to be mindful of balance in your life.

Ask yourself the following questions and journal your responses:

- How can I achieve balance in my work life? What other factors will help me attain balance to perform better at work or enjoy my work more?

____________________________________________________________

____________________________________________________________

____________________________________________________________

____________________________________________________________

- How do I attend to myself and my own needs in my life? How can I do better? What is one thing that I love to do that brings me joy and helps keep me calm? Can I commit to doing at least that one thing 15-20 minutes a day as a way to show myself the love and kindness I deserve?

____________________________________________________________

____________________________________________________________

____________________________________________________________

____________________________________________________________

- How can I get my "Actual Priorities Pie" to look more like my "Balanced Life Pie?" What sacrifices am I willing to make? What things am I not willing to compromise?

- How do I feel when I eat? Do I eat when I feel anxious? What do I eat at those times? Do I eat when I'm depressed? How do I feel like when I'm eating and after I have eaten at these times? Do I eat when I'm not hungry?

- What can I do to take better care of my body?

- On a scale of 1-10 (1 being very little, 10 being a lot), on average, how much stress do I live with?

- What emotions do I experience most often? By looking into them, exploring and understanding them, can I begin to let them be without getting attached and believing my own "story" of me? What kind of messages have I been given in life about the experience and expression of my emotions?

# Chapter Five

## MANAGING YOUR STRESS

The key to reducing your stress is living *with* your life rather than living *against* your life. If you think about it, your life is unfolding minute by minute in a way that is totally out of your control. There are many factors that can change in a second that will alter the course of your life forever: illness, an accident, the death of someone dear to you, hitting the lottery, getting laid off from a job, even the election of political officials, to name a few. These can be positive or negative, but either way, they are out of your control. **Learning to roll *with* your life rather than getting rolled over *by* your life is the key to the healthy balancing of your stress.**

Jon Kabat-Zinn, known for his Mindfulness-Based Stress Reduction (MBSR) program, reminds us to think of our minds as the ocean. Regardless of what is happening at the surface, whether placid on a clear, sunny day, or rolling with high waves brought on by the high winds of a storm, if you were to drop twenty feet below the surface, you would find the water to be quite calm and peaceful. Our minds are also like this. You may be in a really good mood, cruising along without a worry in the world (the clear sunny day at the ocean), or may be barraged with one thing after another that leaves you wondering if things could get any worse (the tempest). Practicing appropriate stress reduction can aid you in being less concerned about what is happening on the ocean surface of your mind, while allowing you to easily access that safe, calm space twenty feet down. When you are there, what is going on at the surface doesn't rattle you as much. You can allow your thoughts and emotions to rise and fall like waves on the ocean while you watch from your safe place below.

Jack Kornfield, a popular author and psychologist, who spent time as a Buddhist monk, encourages us to develop our minds to be like the sky ("Mind Like Sky" on his *Guided Meditations* CD). Regardless of what may travel through the sky (i.e. clouds, storms, planes, meteors), the sky is unaffected and remains constant. Again, the teaching is to allow life's uncontrollable moments to pass into and out of our awareness without allowing yourself to get snared in all the drama.

These are beautiful analogies brought forth by gifted, wise men. I often think of it in a much simpler, probably soon to be outdated way. Maybe this will work for you. Simply ask yourself, "Is it better to *play* pinball or to *be* the pinball?" You can be bounced around in your life by things that happen and your reactions to them, or you can simply observe them for what they are and when all the bouncing around is done, you can go on your way to whatever is next.

Managing your stress is like losing weight. You can go on a crash diet, lose a ton of weight, the program ends, and you wind up right back where you started or worse. This is because you have not adequately dealt with the underlying problem of why you overeat or make poor food choices to begin with. What would serve you better is to make slow, steady, incremental change that works *with* your life, requires relatively little effort, and is sustainable. This is addressed in more detail in the next chapter.

Popular methods people employ to reduce stress such as taking naps, watching television, reading books, listening to favorite music, or working out (when used in an attempt to relieve stress) are like the crash diets above. They may help you take your mind off of your life for a bit, but your life is still there waiting for you when you are done. That is the funny thing about life; as long as you are alive, it is always there. In a way it is like a shadow–you can run from your shadow, but each time you turn, it is still there.

So what I would like to offer you is not an escape *from* your life, but a new way of engaging *with* your life. There are many wonderful methods out there. The important thing is to find what works best for you. The goal is to bring your body, mind, and spirit into alignment, accompanied by an unshakeable sense of stability and inner peace. Once you accomplish this, you will find yourself in a much different relationship with yourself, your health, and your life.

I have mentioned previously the disastrous effects of stress on the body. So many of the common conditions that affect people's health are brought on, at least in part, by unmitigated stress build up. To refresh your memory, these conditions include, but certainly are not limited to, high blood pressure, heart disease, high blood sugar (type II diabetes), poor thyroid function, infections, autoimmune diseases, wound healing difficulties, anxiety, and depression. Stress may even play a role in the development of cancer.

Many people, perhaps due to conditioning (such as growing up in an environment where there was a premium placed on "being tough") automatically suppress and store stress in their body without ever even recognizing it. Others realize it is there, but do not want to bother anyone about it, or feel it is a sign of weakness to express their feelings about it. Let me be the first to tell you if you are in this group, there is no greater sign of strength than acknowledging what is going on inside you, expressing it and letting it be.

Ironically, it is the "being tough" mentality that hurts us the most. Being true to your self, acknowledging what is felt or experienced internally, and letting it out in a healthy way (for instance not by punching a wall or another person) is a show of confidence and inner strength unlike any other. All that is required is for you to truly be yourself. It is sad that this is so hard for us to do, isn't it? Imagine a world where people did this, and the explosive outbursts of stored emotions could be avoided. Maybe *this* is what John Lennon was singing about.

When it comes to management of stress, I advocate a system involving **the 4M's**:

- ***Mindfulness***
- ***Meditation***
- ***Movement***
- ***Massage***

## Mindfulness

Being mindful is to be aware of the present moment, as it is, without judgment. It is cultivated by the other three M's. Mindfulness is a way of life, not any one specific technique. Each moment is born, lives briefly, and is gone, giving way to the next. No two moments are ever the same. We spend so much time and effort in our lives trying to recreate lived moments, certain desired feelings, or to maintain some state of being to which we desperately cling. It does no good, because one of the greatest truths in life is that *everything* is in a constant state of change. This includes our bodies and, thus, our health. There is never any guarantee from one moment to the next what may transpire, so appreciation of life as it is right now is of the utmost importance. Even if you are experiencing pain, realize that this is your body's experience right now, and that this, too, is impermanent. Anything that arises in your body or mind or surroundings, is all part of your journey through life. Take each moment for what it is, acknowledge its significance, and move on.

Nothing is meant to last forever. As much as I would love to keep my two little girls little forever, I can't. No amount of fixation, grasping or control is ever going to change that. In fact, I find that I love the individuals that they are more and more each day. I look forward to each moment as to what one of them may do or say. There is always something new to experience with them that somehow is always more sweet, beautiful, or amazing than whatever was going on just the second before. There is no greater gift you can give yourself or your child than just appreciating him or her for who he or she is at exactly the time you are together.

Imagine your body as your dear friend. Appreciate it in every moment. Listen to what it tells you. Get to know it and allow it to know you. Love it unconditionally. Let it know that no matter what it may ever say, do, or be, that you love it just the same, just as you would your child, mother, best friend, or pet. You are the only you that you will ever be, and your body is the only one you will have in this lifetime. Why is it that we so often treat our pets and plants better than we do our bodies?

Your body is made up of trillions of cells all working together in a precisely orchestrated symphony that allows you to exist, which you usually pay attention to only when something goes wrong. Did you ever have a teacher, coach, or parent who was quick to let you know when you messed up, but never once praised you for anything good you did? Did you ever feel that people only noticed you when you screwed up? I think we have all felt this at some time or another. This is how so many of us treat our bodies. Developing a more loving, forgiving, and compassionate relationship with your body may be the best thing you could ever do for your health, far beyond what any pill, surgery, workout, or diet could ever offer.

Become aware of your breath. Right now as you read this, be aware of the fact that you are breathing. Feel the air as it fills your lungs and leaves again. That breath will never be there again. Your life is made up of a certain number of breaths. The average person breathes about sixteen times per minute. Multiply this by sixty minutes in an hour, then twenty-four hours in a day, 365 days in a year, and then by however many years you may ultimately live. That is the number of breaths you have in this existence. How many of your breaths have you ever sat and noticed? How many times have you turned your full awareness to one single breath. Each breath is one come and gone, like a dotted line on a highway on your journey through life. Take some time each day to focus in on a few breaths. Feel what the air feels like as it passes your nostrils and the warmth of it as it exits. Feel the freshness of the new air entering your body and the positive energy it brings to sustain your life. Feel the release of the toxins on the out breath, purifying your body as they are released. How does this make you feel? Take a moment to close your eyes and really experience this. Master Charles Cannon says, "Breath is life, and life is now." There is perhaps no better way to be connected to the present moment of your life and vitality than through the awareness of your breath.

Your breath can be your anchor in the present moment. When you feel emotions welling up at work, or you are getting frustrated with your child or husband, be aware of your breath, find the present moment, and note what you are feeling in your body, and what thoughts are in your mind. So many times, our emotions are being triggered by events, thoughts, or feelings from long ago, or by fear of something that may result in the future from whatever is going on in this moment. Be aware that the past is gone. It is important as everything that has happened to you, every person you have encountered, every dream that you have had, all that you have ever experienced, has led you to where and who you are right now. For better or worse, the past and all it has entailed is your journey that has brought you to this particular destination that is now. What you do with now will begin to shape what unfolds next. The future has not yet happened. Let go of the need to control it, you can't. No one can. There are infinite numbers of things that could happen in the world in the next moment that could change everything as you currently know it.

Live now. Be present. Choose your life in this second. Love yourself for who you are in this very breath. Your health, happiness, and true fulfillment awaits.

## Meditation

By far the best way for your true self to emerge is through meditation. This is the route by which you begin to de-clutter your mental attic and restore order and understanding to your life. By observing your thoughts, emotions, and the machinations of your ego, you can begin to understand how and why you are the way you are. By observing these aspects of yourself, acknowledging and letting them be, they will start to clear. As this happens, your load will lighten, the "clutter" in your mind will start to dissipate, your body will relax, and you will find your true voice. You may experience openness, creativity, or a general sense of wholeness such as you have never known. People spend so much energy and concentration on what "I want" or what "should be," that they literally wear themselves out. Part of the beauty of meditation is that it allows you to realize that seeking and grasping gets you nowhere. It is actually by letting go of the need to control, surrendering to what is, and allowing layers upon layers of accumulated clutter in your brain to be released that allows you to be open enough to find that which you seek. It is often right in front of or within you from the get-go. You have just been too blinded by conditioning and illusion to see it. The illusions are stories concocted by yourself, your environment, and/or society, that lead you to believe reality is something other than what it is. This includes stories about yourself and who you are. Meditation allows us to cut through illusion and get in touch with what is really important in our lives.

The word "meditation" conjures up many different images for many different people. Meditation can be a formal practice, like that undertaken by Buddhist monks, or can simply be just sitting with yourself in silence for a period of time. For me, it is somewhere in between. One of my favorite tips on meditation comes from Adyashanti who asserts that the key to "true meditation" is in "letting go of the meditator." In other words, don't try too hard, just let it happen. "Rest as awareness," he says. The mirror exercise, the sitting practice, and the breath awareness exercises earlier in the book are all examples of different types of meditation. Meditation basically is some version of quieting the mind, observing what unfolds, redirecting to some focal point (often the breath) and doing this over and over again.

The real benefits of meditation come from repetition. Commit to a daily practice of some sort. Jon Kabat-Zinn in his MBSR program asks for 45 minutes a day, six days a week. I would encourage you to commit to whatever is reasonable for you. I would rather you meditate 15 minutes a day than do nothing. Start with what makes sense for you, and then add time as you are able to do so. Don't sell yourself short; the more time you commit, the greater the potential rewards. It is important, however, to let your experience unfold as it does, and not to seek any particular effect. Have faith in the process. For most people, the experience is so positive that they start seeking more time to practice.

The previously described sitting practice is a great exercise in basic meditation. Sitting with breath awareness as above is also a great place to start. When you begin, set a timer on your phone, i-Pod or alarm clock for 15 minutes. Sit or lie in a comfortable position, close your eyes, and focus your attention on your breathing. Allow it to be as it is. Feel the rise and fall of your belly on the inbreath and outbreath respectively. Do this until the timer goes off. You will find that your mind will wander, but don't get frustrated. The more it wanders, the more you need this practice. Gently note that your mind has wandered, and without judging or being critical of yourself, turn your attention back to the breath. Repeat this as many times as is necessary until the meditation is over. Thank yourself for giving yourself this time and effort, and nourishing yourself in this way. Repeat this exercise daily. Within a relatively short time you will start noticing a shift in yourself. That is because this process actually allows your brain to rewire itself in certain ways that are associated with present moment awareness, redirecting attention and emotional stability.

Walking practice is also good. Try standing on your feet, becoming aware of how they feel on the ground, and how the ground feels under them. Shift your weight to your right foot, then your left. Roll forward on your toes, then back to your heels. Repeat this a few times. When you are ready, slowly lift your right foot, move it forward through the air then gently place your heel down, roll to the toes as the other foot rises and lands. Continue meditating as you walk slowly, noting every sensation in your foot as it glides through the air, strikes the floor then lifts again. Use the fall of your foot to the floor as your focus, as you previously did with your breath. As your mind strays, and it will, gently return your awareness to your feet. Do this for ten to fifteen minutes, and notice how you feel when you are finished. Add more time to the exercise as you become comfortable with it.

The sitting meditation exercise earlier in the book contains a version of the body scan meditation. Try this lying down. Spend a couple of minutes becoming aware of each section of the body, sensing any tension, breathing a few breaths into and out of these areas, then taking a few deep breaths, and releasing the tension from your body. Get a sense of where you tend to hold stress. Let these areas be for now, and watch how they change over time. Note the sensations in each body region. This brings a great deal of awareness of your body, and as I have mentioned previously, awareness is one of the major keys to developing healthy balance in your life.

## Movement

Relax, you do not have to go pound out two hours on the treadmill to move your body in a meaningful way. While cardiovascular exercise is important for your health as well as your emotional well-being, what I am going to focus on here is *mindful movement*. This involves making slow, deliberate movements of your body while maintaining full awareness of the moving part of your body in space. This helps to enhance your moment to moment presence and enhances your overall state of mindfulness. It also is great for improving blood and lymph circulation in your body.

Common types of mindful movement include Hatha yoga, Qi Gong, and Tai Chi, though any movement done slowly with the purpose of enhancing awareness of your body and relaxing your mind will do. Most importantly, move so that you are working within the limits of your body, allowing a gentle stretch, but avoiding pain and injury. This is great for increasing blood flow to your brain, heart, and muscles, and provides a much better workout than you may think. This type of movement is also great at helping release stored muscular tension from stress or from the clearing the emotional residue that may occur as a result of meditation. Meditation gets the tension moving, while movement allows it to be released. In a way it is like having clogged up sinuses: meditation is like the decongestant, while movement is like blowing your nose. Maybe this comparison is a bit graphic and crude, but hopefully you get the point.

Another great way to mindfully move is walking. Walking is great for your cardiovascular health, helps in oxygenating your brain, and also aids with maintaining emotional stability. Go for a walk outside, weather permitting. Start with twenty minutes or so, longer if you wish. Walk just fast enough so that you can still maintain conscious awareness of the rise and fall of each foot as you walk. Breathe in the fresh air. Note the scents that you encounter, and become aware of the trees, flowers, and grass as you pass them. Notice any animals at play. Allow your mind to wander, then gently bring it back to your footfalls or to your breath. Note that everything you see is an expression of life, as are you. Trees grow, eat, drink, excrete, breathe and reproduce just as you and I do. Squirrels care for their young, play and eat just as you and I do. You may notice vibrant colors, scents, rocks, or bushes you have never seen before, despite the fact that you may have driven or walked this path a thousand times. If you happen to be out somewhere at night, stop, take a couple of breaths and look up at the sky. We so often forget about the beauty of the stars above. It never ceases to amaze me how small, yet significant I feel when I contemplate the universe around me. Awareness is a beautiful gift to offer yourself, and it is right here with you, every moment of every day, in every breath you take.

## Massage

The last, but certainly not the least of the 4M's is massage. I throw this in, because massage for me serves a couple of very important purposes when it comes to relieving stress. Like movement, it helps clear areas of held tension or "blockages" to your energy flow as you begin to clear it through meditation and movement. It also is a great way to further your awareness of your body. Feeling areas of soreness or tension while getting massaged will help you gain knowledge of how you carry stress in your muscles. It seems that whatever areas of your body tighten up during a particular event or emotional state, will tighten again when you encounter a similar or related event. Therefore, we tend to hold stress in relatively consistent areas. For me it is up around my left shoulder blade. Where is yours?

Try doing a basic mindful breathing meditation while getting a massage. Better yet, allow the touch of the therapist to be your focusing point. It may be of great interest to you what thoughts or feelings arise as the therapist works a point of tension. I find that memories or feelings often come up, just as if they were stored as a memory in the muscle itself. As they come up, observe them and let them go, just as you do in meditation. They will slowly but surely clear out over time, and you will find yourself less tense or "tight" as time goes on.

If for no other reason, get a massage every once and again to treat yourself to a relaxing experience. You are worth it. Make sure to communicate to your therapist any areas of particular concern or ones on which you would like some extra time spent. It is your massage. Make sure you get the maximum possible benefit from it.

In summary, the key to reducing your stress is being aware of your body, thoughts, and emotions in the present moment, right now as things are happening. Knowing how to observe your inner world without getting caught up in it will allow you to respond to situations rather than reacting. Mindfulness allows you to get out of your autopilot mode and to once again be in the driver's seat of your life. By being aware of your true thoughts and feelings, and learning to respond to them appropriately you can enjoy *playing* pinball and stop *being* the pinball.

Ask yourself the following questions, then journal your responses:

- How can I be more present in my life?

- Where in my body do I feel tension when I feel sad? Angry? Lonely? Down in the dumps?

- How can I incorporate the 4 M's in my life?

- When was the last time I treated myself to a truly relaxing experience?

- Where is the closest place I can get a massage asap?

Recommended Reading:

| | |
|---|---|
| Thich Nhat Hanh | *The Miracle of Mindfulness*<br>*You Are Here* |
| Jon Kabat-Zinn | *Full Catastrophe Living*<br>*Wherever You Go, There You Are*<br>*Mindfulness for Beginners* (contains guided meditation CD) |
| Bob Stahl and Elisha Goldstein | *A Mindfulness-Based Stress Reduction Workbook* (this has a great guided meditations CD also) |

CDs/Downloads regarding Meditation:

| | |
|---|---|
| Adyashanti | "True Meditation" |
| Pema Chodron | "How to Meditate" |
| Rick Hanson | "Stress Proof Your Brain" |
| Jon Kabat-Zinn | "Guided Mindfulness Meditation" (includes the body scan 2 yoga routines and the sitting practice) |
| Jack Kornfield | "Meditation for Beginners"<br>"Guided Meditations for Self-Healing" |

DVDs for movement:

Body Wisdom Media "Yoga for Beginners and Beyond"
(Three DVDs, you pick your level and length of time – DVDs include one set of routines for stress relief and one for inflexible people. It is very good and quite doable for anyone – my eight year old daughter does them with me)

Lee Holden "Qi Gong for Self-Healing"

The Arthritis Foundation also has a "Tai Chi for Arthritis" DVD you can order from their website.

## Chapter Six

# NOURISHING YOUR BODY, MIND AND SPIRIT

The preceding chapters of this book are about learning to be okay with yourself as you are right now in the present moment and for every subsequent moment that arises. Whatever your judgments about yourself may be, the fact is, right now you are exactly as you are. This chapter is about taking good care of who you are in an effort to be the best version of you that you can be. That is kind of a tongue twister. Read it again carefully. You are the only you that you will ever be. It is best to learn to be the best at being you that you can, rather than constantly trying to be something else (remember the ego?).

Caring for yourself is the greatest gift you can give yourself as well as all others in your life. The notion that attending to your own needs is somehow selfish is inappropriate, outdated, and flat-out wrong. So let's just do away with it. Good, that was easy…I feel much better now, how about you?

You see, if you are constantly attending to others but never to yourself, you will wear down, get exhausted, grumpy, and sick. Any time you do have to yourself, you will spend feeling guilty and ruminating about all the things you "should be" doing for someone else. You will be stressed, which will lead to further exhaustion, poor digestion, fatigue, and illness. Anxiety and depression will set in and off you go. The same thing goes if you are always worried about what everyone else thinks of you. This has been a major issue for me. No matter what you do in life, there will always be someone who is unsatisfied with it.

You will constantly ruminate about what you should have said, done, worn, or whatever. How can you ever be at peace if this is your main concern? It is my goal to help you put a stop to this. The fact is, as Pema Chodron says, you are "perfect just as you are."

I am not saying that you should not be helpful or unavailable to people in your life–quite the opposite. But, if you are adequately addressing your own needs and taking care of yourself, you will be in a much better place to lend a hand, will be more clear, focused, and strong when you do, and will have less resentments about it.

> **So, recapping the entire message of this book: Find balance in your life, reduce your level of stress, and take good care of yourself.** Seems simple, right? It turns out, not so much. But you *are* on the right path. Read on.

Now that you are consciously working on finding balance in your life and are becoming more effective at being less stressed, now it is time to learn how to deepen your level of health, well-being, and satisfaction in your life. Nourishing yourself head to toe and beyond is your next endeavor.

## Body

In our society, we are obsessed with our bodies. Frankly, our obsession is out of control. Let us agree that our bodies come in all shapes, sizes, heights, weights, hair colors, skin colors, bra sizes, intellectual levels, and with the full range of facial wrinkles, skin blemishes, and athletic abilities. There is beauty in this diversity. I love that we are not all the same. How boring would it be if we all looked and acted exactly alike? As my dad always says, "If we all liked the same things, there would only be vanilla ice cream and black cars."

Nourishing your body is not about starving or fattening or shaping it to a certain something you want to be. It is about taking good care of the one you have, whatever shape or size it may have currently taken. Genetically, we are all different, and therefore have different needs. There is not one "perfect" way to be or look. There is only looking like you look. Wanting to be something else is always the work of the ego. It likes to tell you "if only you looked like that" or "wore that size" or "had those boots" you would be happy. The true self just wants to express itself as it is. It also wants to be happy and healthy. Remember, the further apart the ego is from the true self, the more unhappiness you will experience. When your ego stops grasping at something else and becomes content in who you currently are, it comes in line with your true self, and you will be happy and content.

Having said that, there are three main aspects to nourishing your body: feeding it, moving it, and loving it. In fact, these three also are critical for the mind and spirit as well. Nourish your body in these ways, and it will find its natural shape. You will look and feel better than you ever have, and you will be healthier to boot. Sounds too good to pass up, doesn't it?

## Feeding your Body

There is much written and published about the feeding of your body. You can't turn on the television, radio, or internet, open a newspaper or magazine, or drive down the street without encountering some piece of information about it. There is always some new fad diet, exercise program, or wonder drug that promises you the body you have always wanted. I would like to save you a lot of time, money, and frustration by letting you in on a little secret. It is much easier and effective to engage yourself in learning to love the body you have, and treating it as such. It does take some time and effort to attend to, but so do your plants, pets, and automobiles. It costs no money and is a relationship that will literally last you a lifetime. Whereas your plants, pets, and cars will come and go in your lifetime, your body is yours for the duration. It is truly with you in good times and bad, in sickness and health, "'til death do you part." So, let's talk about how to take care of it.

Most of the problems you likely encounter with food are not as much in what you are eating, rather in how, when, and why you are eating. Understanding these factors is first and foremost. How do you do this? Did you say, "Awareness?" if so, you are catching on. Try the following exercise at least one meal a day, then more often if you can. It will become second nature after a while.

- Before preparing food or eating, close your eyes, take three to five deep breaths and feel your level of hunger. Rate your hunger on a scale of one to ten (one being starving, ten being stuffed). Never let yourself go below a four or eat yourself over an eight (comfortable, but not "full"). See if you can figure out why you are eating. Are you eating because your body is truly hungry, or are you eating to "feel" better or different? Are you having any cravings? Most overeating in our society is emotional overeating (i.e. drowning one's sorrows in ice cream, or "treating" yourself to a brownie because "I deserve it"). This on occasion is okay, but should not be used as an excuse to eat foods your adult brain is telling you not to eat at this particular moment. "Mental" hunger cannot be satisfied. This is why it is so important to understand the messages of your own body. Eat until you are satisfied (a seven or eight on the hunger scale), then stop. In general, you need smaller portions than you are likely used to. Avoid seconds.

- When you eat, just eat. Avoid eating while driving, watching television, reading or while you are involved in other distracting behaviors. Engaging in other activities while eating leads to overeating because you don't notice when you have had enough. You should really be able to taste your food and appreciate what you are eating, and see what feelings develop in your body and mind while eating. This leads to a sense of true nourishment, and you will find that you are more satisfied and will tend to eat less than you would eat if you were not giving your full attention to your food.

- Use slow steady breaths prior to and during eating. This serves to calm the body and aid with digestion. When the body is stressed, the digestive process is slowed or shut down, as is absorption. This leads to a continued sense of hunger despite having eaten an adequate amount. Reflux is a common side effect of this.

- Take one bite at a time, noticing the food in your mouth and the flavors and sensations associated with it. Do not load your fork or spoon until you have chewed and swallowed the previous bite. Make sure to take long, deep, slow breaths during eating. Also drink plenty of water and also try warm liquids such as hot tea with meals. This helps you digest your food and avoid overeating. Better digestion means that you are getting what you need out of your food, and you will feel more satisfied with less food and will be less likely to overeat.

- After your meal, again, take 3-5 deep breaths with eyes closed and notice how your stomach and body feel. Write down briefly what thoughts or feelings you experienced during your meal; you may learn a lot.

When you eat is also important. Avoid eating at times of stress, and take a few minutes to mindfully breathe and allow tension to clear as much as possible. You will avoid emotional eating (eating to satisfy an emotional need rather than a nutritional one), and will digest more efficiently and completely. Eat a satisfying breakfast and a smaller dinner. Make lunch the main meal of the day as your body digests best in the middle of the day (when the sun is at its peak). Be aware of your surroundings and the food on your plate. Avoid "inhaling" your food (known as conditioned overeating), and eat slowly, enjoy your company if you have some, and savor every bite–your relationship with food will start to improve. Also, be mindful to not eat within two hours of your bedtime as digestion is slowest at this time. If you do, you may have more difficulty sleeping well, have issues with reflux, and will tend to gain more weight than if you don't eat in this time period.

As far as *what* to eat, I tend to think of this as simply as possible. Eat plenty of fruits and vegetables, as close to the way they came out of the ground or off the tree as possible. Prepare vegetables by steaming, roasting, or sautéing them in peanut, grapeseed, or other neutral oil, or eat them raw. Organic dairy, produce, and meats are good to avoid hormones, pesticides, and other toxic chemicals that can be harmful to your body. Beans, natural nut butters, and lean meats are a good source of protein. Choose whole grain pastas and multigrain breads and cereals when possible. Avoid food items that contain high-fructose corn syrup (be careful, it is everywhere), trans fats, refined sugars and flour, or anything that is individually wrapped at room temperature (highly processed). One friend of mine once said, "So just avoid the middle of the grocery store." Whatever works best for you, do it.

There are no inherently "good" and "bad" foods. These types of terms often lead us to view ourselves as "good" or "bad" for eating them. Think of foods as being "nutritious," "non-nutritious," or "neutral." You will judge yourself less and have a healthier relationship with food already. Stay off the scale. The stress of constantly checking your weight and the disappointment of not having lost the right amount of weight or at having gained some perpetuate the chronic stress response, making you more likely to gain rather than lose. Be aware, listen to your body, and eat to nourish yourself, period. If you have the occasional dessert, remember, it is all about balance, not to say that having a piece of cake then starving yourself for three days is appropriate; it isn't. Continue to be aware, focus on reducing your stress, and follow the tips above. Your body will do the rest. There will be no need to check the scale. Your body will find the shape for which it is programmed and the way you look and feel will tell the story. If you must gauge your relationship with food, check your weight every 3-4 months. Your weight, once stabilized in this way, should never fluctuate more than 5-7 pounds. If it does, re-read the above exercise and continue on.

Most importantly, if you do forget everything I have just told you, overeat, or even outright binge, don't be harsh on yourself. Smile, forgive yourself, and start over. This moment has passed and a new beginning awaits in the next. Just as in meditation when you direct your attention from your wandering mind back to your breath, direct your focus back to the task at hand and be kind to yourself. This embodies the mindful approach to life. Just the fact that you are now paying attention is a big step. Remember, it is okay for change to be gradual, as it is more likely to last this way.

## Moving Your Body

I don't have much to add after the discussion on movement in the last chapter. Move mindfully, walk outside when possible, and pay attention to your body. Our bodies are made to move in a certain way.

Be as kind to your body in movement as you are in feeding it. Anything you are doing and you think "I probably shouldn't be doing this," you are probably right. Aches and pains can be a sign of impending or actual injury. Note what hurts. If certain sensations present themselves as "the usual" after exercise, let them be. If something "unusual" occurs, or the usual fails to respond in its typical fashion, you should see your doctor.

If it is more intensive cardiovascular exercise you seek, then, as an orthopedic surgeon, I would recommend elliptical machines, walking briskly, stationary bicycling, or anything done in water. These exercises are great for maintaining healthy muscles, bones, and joints, while limiting harmful wear and tear. Get your heart rate up somewhere in the 100-120 beats per minute range for 30 minutes or so 3-4 times per week. It is always best to check with your physician before beginning any new exercise program.

## Loving Your Body

Sadly, for most people, this is the toughest of the three. We are under constant pressure to "get in shape" or to be somehow different than we are. You know my feelings on this. While it is important to be kind to yourself and be healthy, it is not important whether you are a size 4, 14, or 24. It is more important that you are the size that is right for you.

If you are making yourself miserable in order to continue fitting yourself into your most beloved pair of jeans, then choose to love yourself as you are, treat your body kindly, and consider buying a new pair of jeans. If you are gaining weight because you are abusing yourself with food and lack of movement, then choose to love your body, allow it to return to its "happy place" and live accordingly. **I cannot emphasize this enough: Your body wants to be happy and healthy; you just have to get out of your own way and let it happen.**

There are as many unhappy, depressed size zeros as size 30s. Don't get caught in the trap that you will be happier if you are thinner. Don't try to be someone else's size, because that person may naturally be that size, or may be just as miserable as you in an effort to maintain it. Be true to yourself, and allow yourself to feel good. Love yourself for who you are, right now, today. Appreciate your body for all the wonderful, simply amazing things it does for you without you ever even knowing it. Love it, care for it, and appreciate it, and it will treat you kindly in return.

In the event you have a serious illness, I can tell you that one of the most inspiring things that I encounter as a cancer specialist are the individuals who come to the realization that their bodies never wanted to become sick; it just happened. Some are even able to make friends with their disease and learn very important lessons by listening to what it and their bodies have to say. Regardless of your situation, it is your situation. For whatever reason, your journey through life has come to this point. The human body is amazing, but not perfect.

Oddly enough, terminal illness has a way of snapping people into a state of mindfulness and, with it, a whole new appreciation of all the little things that mean so much. I see it all the time. Don't wait to be on your death bed to stop and take a look around. As Jon Kabat-Zinn says, "Every day you wake up there is a lot more right with you than wrong." Life is happening every second, in every breath. It is there to be taken in and enjoyed right now. In fact, your whole life is right now, over and over and over again. At some point it will be over, but not right now. Your body is breathing for you, your heart pumping, your brain processing, every second of every day, without rest. As you sleep, your body continues working to keep you alive. Love it, thank it, appreciate it. Let it know you care. It is a choice you'll never regret.

## Mind

Your mind can be your best friend or your worst enemy. Mark Twain said, "Some of the worst things in my life never happened." We tend to create so many stories about ourselves and other people's judgments or thoughts about us, it can be utterly exhausting. It is therefore of the utmost importance to nourish your mind, to ultimately allow it to be free from all of the clutter that makes you miserable. An open, free, clear mind is relaxed, creative and expansive. I think we have all had the experience where you struggle and struggle to remember something, a phone number for instance. The second you stop thinking about it and move on, it suddenly pops into your mind. Imagine if your whole life were spent in that moment of clarity where things just came to you, without all the struggling. Would you believe that you, just as you are today, can achieve this?

## Feeding Your Mind

The mind, like the body, needs food, hence the term "food for thought." This is true in the literal and the figurative sense. Have you ever noticed how hard it is to concentrate when you are very hungry? Have you also noticed how hard it is to stay awake when you are stuffed? Your brain needs food to function. A balanced life and a nourishing diet are necessary for your mind to work properly. I will defer to Dr. Mark Hyman on the gritty details (see below). Suffice it to say, eat well, minimize toxins that affect your brain (excessive alcohol, drugs, cigarettes, heavy metals such as lead and mercury), and keep your stress and anxiety levels under control. Your mind will work much better.

The mind also needs to be fed intellectually. I talked in the "Balance" chapter about stimulating the brain. This is important. Your brain needs to be exercised just like your body. This overlaps with the "movement" part of this discussion, but the message is to find a way to continue learning throughout your entire life. Do puzzles, challenge yourself at work, read, do something new. Your mind needs to be fed knowledge, memories, and information. There is nothing sadder to me than a physically healthy person with little to no remaining cognitive function. Appreciate your mind for the fact that it is there. Clear your head by practicing mindfulness and reducing your stress. Allow your mind to work with you rather than against you. Listen to your mind and feed it. It will tell you—just listen.

## Moving Your Mind

Just as moving your body is important in relieving tension, so it is for your mind. Exercising your mind is quite the opposite of moving your body. Whereas moving your body involves engaging in activity above and beyond what is required for most of your daily activities, exercising the mind involves quieting it down; by that I mean meditation.

Daniel Siegel and Richard Davidson, among others, have published quite a bit on the positive effects of mindfulness meditation on the functioning of the brain. It turns out, while your experience during meditation may be subtle, there is a lot of activity going on upstairs. Just the process of redirecting the mind back to the breath from its wanderings into thought is quite helpful in the process of maintaining emotional equilibrium and maintaining present moment awareness at times when it would be easiest to just react. The amount of rewiring that your brain goes through and the effectiveness of it directly correlate with the amount of time spent in meditative practice. Remember though, that as little as 10-15 minutes every day or every other day can be enough to have a significant impact. Becoming aware of the musings of your mind goes a long way toward reducing your anxiety, calming the chronic stress response, and thus improving your overall state of health and well-being.

Once you have exercised your brain through meditation, then put it to use. Integrating what you are learning is the best way to make it stick. One of the best descriptions I have seen of how to do this is in Diane Rizzetto's book *Waking Up to What You Do*. She tells of a young trapeze artist who says that the moment where the bar stops swinging in one direction and starts going the other is where the trick is born, and it's called the "dead spot." Rizzetto goes on to describe the dead spots that occur in our lives. There are major ones like a job change, the end of a relationship, or death of a loved one. But there are also the ones that occur in a split second. These are the ones that are so difficult, because they come and go before you know what happened.

Usually, the situation is that someone says something and you react. Later you may feel bad about it, or maybe wish you had said something more. But catching yourself in that "dead spot" between the spot where the action has occurred and your reaction begins and choosing your response as opposed to allowing your autopilot to knee-jerk can make a huge difference in the outcome. I can tell you from countless encounters with patients and other physicians, if your ego comes out to play, more often than not, so will theirs. As Ram

Dass says, "What you meet in another being is the projection of your own level of evolution."

Identifying the welling up of emotion and the reaction that is coming before you fire it out there, recognizing it for what it is and choosing a more skilled response gives you a much better chance at your true self engaging the other person's true self and having a much healthier interchange for it. Sometimes it is as simple as just being 100 percent honest, no matter how hard it may be. The other person may get it or not; that is not your responsibility. It is only your responsibility to be true to yourself. How the other person reacts or responds is up to him. The chips will fall where they fall.

An example might be if a co-worker were to start disparaging another colleague for being lazy. You might normally get caught and agree or listen to the story and immediately assume your co-worker's account to be the truth. The fact is, you don't know the truth of the situation, since your co-worker can only see it through his own eyes. Who knows what really happened? In the "dead spot" you know this to be true, and you may choose to not respond at all, say that you don't really know the individual, or come to his defense if you know that laziness is not a particular characteristic of that person. Your co-worker's ego needs that individual to be seen as lazy, whether he is or is not. Your ego doesn't need to get involved. Your true self may feel compassion for both individuals, recognizing the insecurity or pain of your co-worker who needs to engage in this type of gossip, and the disparaged individual for being the target of this venom. By choosing the more skilled response, you have avoided further escalation of this rhetoric.

You can probably see how this may be much more difficult if you were being directly confronted. By choosing to allow your ego to stay at home, you can confront maliciousness with humility and disarm it right away. Also, I would warn you that the ego loves to project our own fear or anger on to others and then respond in kind. The other, in fact, may not have had any fear or anger to begin with, but now you have introduced it into the mix. Observe your "dead spots." See if you can start to delay your knee-jerk reactions to situations long enough to choose the response you want. You may still be angry, and it may be perfectly appropriate, but choosing this response is much healthier than reacting with anger without knowing why. The "dead spot" can only start to be identified after present-moment awareness has been cultivated through mindfulness meditation.

## Loving Your Mind

This can also be tough. As with the body, our mind is what our mind is. While you may wish it were something else or like someone else's, it isn't. It is yours for the long haul. Many of your processes and thought patterns that go on are the result of early childhood learning and conditioning, for better or worse. You may or may not be able to change these patterns, but you can learn to observe them, and not allow them to be in control.

The key to learning to love your mind is compassion, compassion for yourself. Through meditation you can learn to observe the movement of your thoughts and come to understand the associated emotions. Emotions are almost always an expression of an underlying thought, even when the thought may not be so apparent. By learning to be compassionate toward your mind, not taking your thoughts and feelings personally, but seeing them for what they are, you will move into a new realm of inner peace. You will realize that everyone has thoughts and feelings not unlike yours. Whatever you are going through, you are not alone. Befriend your mind; listen to what it is telling you. Be your own best friend and pay attention to your inner dialogue. You will catch your ego and true self communicating. It can be quite bizarre the first time one experiences this. Don't buy into your own stories, simply find them amusing and let them go. It can be quite disarming to practice this. Like the body movement, you will start to feel the tension slowly releasing from your body. Your body, mind, and health will thank you.

## Spirit

Your spirit is your very essence. It is that force or energy that animates your body. It is the purest form of your true self. So how does one go about nourishing that? In a word, love. Love can take many forms and mean something very different to each individual. It is personal, diverse and yet, universal. Ram Dass teaches that the smallest particle linking everything in the universe together is love. It *is* who we are. Regardless of your spiritual or religious background, this belief is common to all of them. Be love and you will receive love. Feed it by being it. Move it by exercising compassion, empathy, and forgiveness. Love your spirit by loving yourself.

There are many descriptions, illustrations, and philosophies about what love is. Never have I seen this soul-level love so beautifully described as in Ram Dass' *Be Love Now*. If you have ever given of yourself, purely out of your own generosity and not for anything expected in return, you have had a taste of it. I remember the first time I laid eyes on my firstborn daughter. I was instantly transformed. I knew all I needed to know about love right then. She would never need to be or do anything other than exactly who she is and I would give anything for her at any moment without hesitation, never asking anything in return. Pure, true, unconditional love at first sight. Then I experienced it all over again with the birth of my other daughter. Unbelievable to me is the heart's ability to open and expand when you allow love to flow unrestricted.

But love isn't always easy. Sometimes, the greatest gift of love is saying "no" or confronting the individual. Allowing someone you care about to persistently destroy himself in front of your eyes without saying or doing anything for fear of "hurting his feelings" or "running him off" is not love. Love is courageous. Love is strong, and occasionally, love is fierce.

This also applies to yourself. Be kind and compassionate to yourself. When you need a kick in the tail, do it in a way that doesn't diminish or demean yourself. Forgive yourself. But most important in all of this…feel. Feel happiness, feel pain, feel sadness, feel loss, feel unending gratitude, feel pride, and feel rejection. Feel it all. It is feeling that makes us human. By feeling what is real for you in the moment, looking into it rather than away from it, and truly experiencing every ounce of it, you allow your soul to breathe. You experience your true self exactly as it is.

By looking your emotions in the face, you can process them appropriately, learn and grow from them, and move on. Boxes don't get stored in your mental attic. Running away from your emotions allows them to pile up one on top of the other until the weight of them literally starts to weigh you down. You experience this as pain, tension, depression, sleep disturbance, or general breakdown of your health. Love yourself enough to be honest, open, and real with yourself. Feel what you feel in exactly the moment you feel it. Confront it head on, and bask in the sensation of it so you can experience exactly what it is to be alive as you–the only you there has ever been and will ever be. It is so beautiful, yet so neglected in our society. Open your heart, clear your mind and reclaim your life.

Try the following exercise as a way to nourish your spirit.

- Sit comfortably, legs planted firmly on the ground, arms untensed, hands resting in your lap. Close your eyes, relax your jaw, and turn your attention to your breath. Again, just notice that you are breathing, and feel the rise and fall of each breath as it happens. When your mind wanders, gently bring it back to the breath. Do this for 3-5 minutes or until you're relaxed, yet aware.

- Next, turn your awareness to your heart area in the center or center-left of your chest. Continue being aware of your breath, but feel as if you're breathing into and out of the heart area. Note what sensations, thoughts, and feelings come up and return your attention to your heart area.

- After a couple of minutes, start with the following mantras. Say them silently, in your mind, one at a time, each on its own inbreath. On the outbreath breathe out any tension or resistance. Note the still point between outbreath and inbreath, then think of the next one on the inbreath.

  "May I be safe."
  "May I be healthy."
  "May I be peaceful."
  "May I know the ease of well-being".

Try a couple of cycles of this with a break of a few breaths in between, and note how you feel.

- When you are ready, do the same, but this time, picture a "positive" person, someone for whom you feel gratitude. Do a couple of cycles of this just as above.

- Next, repeat the mantras for a "neutral" person. This may be an acquaintance or someone you see regularly, but have no particular personal relationship with.

- Next, pick a "difficult" person. This is someone who has caused you pain, or who you have a very hard time forgiving for past wrongs. Note the feelings that arise with this one. Allow a couple minutes of breathing after, noticing your thoughts and feelings, and bringing attention back to your breathing in the heart area. You may choose to bring the focus back to yourself and repeat the mantras to re-center if this person was particularly challenging for you.

- Finally, repeat the mantras as previously, but for all people.

- Spend a couple of minutes in breathing awareness. Note how the heart area feels. Note any emotions, thoughts, or sensations you feel. When you're ready, open your eyes. Journal how you feel, and any particular positive or negative thoughts and emotions that may have arisen. This is an example of a traditional "lovingkindness," or Metta meditation. Mix this into your meditation practice every once in a while and notice how your experience changes over time. I would encourage you to personalize your mantras as you get comfortable, so they are more meaningful to you.

Ask yourself the following questions and journal your responses:

- How can I change the way I eat to provide a more nourishing experience?

____________________________________________

____________________________________________

____________________________________________

____________________________________________

- What kinds of food do I eat when I'm stressed?

- How can I incorporate meaningful movement of my body into my daily routine?

- What kinds of images, positive or negative, do I have about my body? Are they true? What is my frame of reference? How did these judgments come to be?

- What do I currently do to nourish my mind? My spirit? How can I make this a priority in my life?

- How am I feeling now compared to when I started this book?

Recommended Reading:

| | |
|---|---|
| Barry Boyce, Ed. | *Mindfulness Revolution* |
| Ram Dass | *Be Love Now* |
| Marc David | *Nourishing Wisdom*<br>*Slow Down Diet* |
| Mark Hyman | *Ultramind Solution* |
| Roger Jahnke | *The Healer Within* |
| Sharon Salzberg | *Lovingkindness Meditation* |
| Daniel Siegel | *The Mindful Brain Mindsight* |

## Chapter Seven

# THE ROLE OF MEDICATION AND SURGERY

Now we have come full circle, back to your interface with the medical system. So far, you have learned how to identify the voice of your true self, clean out all the stored garbage of the ego in your mental attic, accept yourself as you are, reduce your stress by use of the 4 M's, and attend to your body, mind, and spirit in a nourishing way. As you practice and integrate all of this into your life, you may feel better than you have in years. You may really start to feel like the you that you remember from your childhood. Now why on Earth would you need a doctor?

First, make sure to make the most of your wellness checks and always attend to your cancer screenings. Even the finest, most luxurious of cars still need maintenance work every now and then. So it is with the body and mind. Your health is precious, and you can never be too careful. And, as much as I hate to say it, **no matter how healthy and well-adjusted you are, you at times will still get ill.** In this regard the answer is simple; see the doctor when you *need* to see the doctor, and go to the hospital when you *need* to go to the hospital. As you deepen your practice with mindfulness, your present-moment awareness of your body will sharpen. Listen to your body's messages; it will tell you when something is wrong. If that signal comes, attend to it, address it, and do what it takes to get through it. If you notice a mass or any pain that is unusual for you, get it checked out. It is much better to be safe than sorry, and regardless of how you may feel about it, you are not "wasting" anyone's time. Approach your encounters with the healthcare system as you would a nice, long, sit-down meal with your closest family or friends (rather than rushing through the drive-thru). Engage, interact, ask questions, and get answers. Express what you need to express, and you will feel fulfilled when your encounter is complete.

Once you have tapped into the healing capacity of an open heart and a clear mind, you can fine-tune your body with the necessary medications or operations to keep the engine running as smoothly as possible. You will also be dialed in to the effects of medications on your body. These may be positive, negative, or neutral. Note what happens when you begin taking a new medication and communicate this to your provider. If you are not sure about something, ask. Remember, this is the only body you will ever have in this lifetime, so treat it kindly.

If and when the time comes for surgery, if your stress is under control, you will be in a more optimized state of healing no matter what your current overall health status may be. Just by attending to the 4 M's and making balance a priority in your life, you will be able to reduce your risk of wound healing problems, infections, and secondary complications from your operation. This does not mean that they cannot or will not happen, because they certainly may, but if they do, you will be much better prepared to handle them.

Being in the hospital can be stressful on many levels in and of itself. Continuing some kind of meditation practice in the hospital can help alleviate this stress and keep you in the present moment. It is often when our minds run away with all the things that could happen, "should" happen, or that are out of our control that things get a bit crazy. Taking some time to focus on your breath when you feel these thoughts coming on, and to nourish your mind and spirit in this way can make your hospital experience as stress-free as possible.

You also may encounter all kinds of thoughts, feelings, and emotions as you meditate. Remember, you are clearing out stored items from your "attic." Hopefully, you will find that you feel lighter and become free of this stored tension. However, depending on your particular path through life, some of the items may be painful or even seemingly unbearable. If this happens, get help. There are many wonderful therapists out there who can help you sort through this time in a healthy fashion. This is very important if you hope to avoid further cluttering of your mental attic. There seems to be sort of a stigma about seeking assistance from a mental health professional, though I believe this to be less so in this day and age than in years past. There really should be no stigma. Many more people than you could possibly imagine see therapists all the time. If you need one, find one with whom you feel comfortable and get to work.

Bottom line...take care of yourself. If you have grasped some of the concepts in this book and made any of them a part of your daily life, you will engage the system appropriately. Pay attention to your body and mind, attend to needs that arise, be as geared up for healing as you can be, and feel better than you have in years.

Chapter Eight

# YOUR LIFE NOW

First off, take a moment to congratulate yourself for getting to this point. It is a distinct act of courage to read a book like this, and you should view it as such. I truly hope the journey for you to this point has been eye-opening. Gaining insight into the inner workings of yourself can be quite interesting, if not outright liberating. So where do you go from here?

As you become more and more familiar with the principles and practices presented in this book, the next step is integrating them into your life. Hopefully, you have already started that process. If so, you have probably found that relatively little change is necessary to accomplish this. Really, most of what is required is a commitment to cultivating a new relationship with yourself and a shift in your perception of your self, life, and circumstances, but this is a very real shift, and should not involve simply telling yourself your life is anything other than exactly what it is.

Regardless of how involved you get with all of this, I would encourage you to adopt at least some of the practices mentioned. It could be as simple as gifting yourself with 30-60 minutes a day of sitting silently and directing your attention inward. As you get more comfortable, you can expand this as suits you. Whatever you choose to do, it needs to work with your life and be sustainable. Remember to keep it in balance though, since life is meant to be lived. The key is to start somewhere. Changes will start to occur and you will start to notice a difference in how you relate to your life. You will likely want to increase the amount of time spent in meditation and/or meditative movement once this becomes apparent.

Also, feel free to experiment. There are many wonderful resources out there to help you in your quest to become happier, healthier, and more fulfilled. Traditional bookselling websites have a multitude of books on meditation, yoga, Qi Gong, and healing yourself from within. Many websites are full of resources as well. If you really get into meditation you may want to get cushions or other supplies. Whatever your practice, living a more mindful life is quite rewarding. It will infiltrate all aspects of your life and render it more satisfying. You will be more engaged with your children, spouse, co-workers, family, friends, and everyone else you encounter. You will begin to understand that nothing anyone else does is directed personally at you. People are all the same, but are at different levels of emotional progression, and therefore are only working with the tools they have. Forgive them for this. Be kind, be mindful and keep smiling with the joy, love, and compassion that is your true nature. It is contagious. People will treat you differently. You will find that people will tend to treat you the way you present yourself to them. If you are defensive and tense, people will tend to respond to you in kind. If you are open, peaceful, and stable, that is what you will see from them. It is rare to encounter a real jerk if you are in a genuinely peaceful place. And if you do, realize that it is his own pain and internal void speaking via his ego, not his true self, and there is certainly no need to take his behavior personally.

It is our unawareness and our states of grasping and control that lead us to suffering and unhappiness, which take their toll on our health and state of well-being. Their collective effects have tremendous harmful impact on our healthcare system, society, and the world at large. Any time you encounter conflict or tension with another individual, be reminded that this is an act of ego on one or both of your parts. Expressing discontent is okay but it is not okay to discount or subvert your own needs for the benefit of someone else. However, if you are aware of what is going on in your head and your body, you will be able to discern what is real and what is your ego reacting. If your ego reacts and you realize this is happening or has happened, forgive yourself, love yourself for being you, and start again. Apologize when necessary. This is the life of mindfulness.

Remember to nourish yourself, spend time in reflection, and move your body to release tension. One thing I do with my daughters is to turn on some good dance music and we "jump around like wild people." This is one way to dance like nobody's watching. Just move your body however feels natural, be spontaneous, and let go. It is a great way to blow off steam, have fun, let loose, and bond with your kids, friends, and family, or, if you are feeling really frisky, try it by yourself.

Finally, *be* just for the sake of being. When you read, just read. When you shower, just shower. Feel the water hit and run down your body. Notice the movement of your hands to the various parts of your body as you wash them. Hear the sounds of the water hitting the floor. Your day will unfold as it unfolds. Focus on the present moment. Have faith that everything right now is exactly as it should be. Be true to your real self. Be yourself, not what you think someone else wants or needs you to be. Express yourself. You are uniquely you, and we are blessed on this planet to have you here, just as you are. Be aware that everyone and everything you encounter is just another expression of life that is the same as you. Feel connected to your world and all that is around you. You are unique, but not an island unto your own. Love and be loved. Forgive and be forgiven. Live just to be alive. Be compassionate. Feel. Live. Breathe. Eat. Move. Relax. Awaken. Life is yours to live, now go and live it!

# Notes

# Notes